What the Bible Says About COVID-19

Are worldwide pandemics foretold in Scripture?

MIKE SMITH

What the Bible Says About COVID-19

Are worldwide pandemics foretold in Scripture?

Pilgrim's Press
PilgrimsPress.com
Admin@PilgrimsPress.com

Library of Congress Control Number: 2019906734

ISBN: 978-1-7323773-0-1 (ebook)
ISBN: 978-1-7323773-1-8 (softcover)
ISBN: 978-1-7323773-2-5 (library binding)
ISBN: 978-1-7323773-3-2 (audio)

Printed in the United States of America

Publisher's Cataloging-In-Publication Data
Name: Smith, Mike, 1952
Title: What the Bible Says About COVID-19
Description: [Ardmore, Oklahoma]: [Pilgrim's Press], [2020]
Identifiers: ISBN 9781732377301 (ebook)
ISBN 9781732377318 (softcover)
ISBN 9781732377325 (library binding)

Subjects: LCSH: Bible Prophecy — Eschatology | Christian Rapture
Classification: LCC BT877 .S65 2019 (ebook) | LCC BT877 (print)
DDC 236.9 — dc23

Scriptures quoted herein are from the King James Version of the Bible, and/or the author's paraphrase thereof; public domain.

Contents

Introduction

When asked, "*What shall be the sign of thy coming, and of the end of the age?* Jesus replied, "*Nation shall rise against nation, and kingdom against kingdom: and there shall be famines, earthquakes, fatal diseases . . . All these are the beginning of sorrows"* (Matthew 24:7-8). In other words, things are going to get worse, much worse, as we approach the end of the age.

Some argue there have always been famines, earthquakes, wars, and diseases. So how are these a sign? Jesus said these things are like birth pains. And any woman that's ever given birth can attest that the pain gets more and more intense, and more frequent, right before the baby pops out. Of course, the baby in this case represents the second coming of Christ.

Many think the second coming and the rapture of the Church are the same, but they're not. These are two separate events. Separate with many distinctions. At the rapture, Christ comes *for* His Church whereas, at the second coming, He comes *with* His Church. At the rapture, our Lord is seen by relatively few whereas, at the second coming, *everyone* sees Him.

These two events are separated by a seven-year period known as the tribulation. That's when there'll be a repeat of the current crisis, another pandemic with a different disease, along with earthquakes and tsunamis, persecution and torture, severe drought, mass starvation, nuclear war, and the list goes on.

Concerning that time, Jesus said there will be a great tribulation, such as the world has never known. Life on Earth will become unbearable, a living nightmare. Sounds dismal at best. Dismal and bleak, very bleak. But the good news is that Christians won't be here.

Before the Antichrist takes over, before God pours out His wrath on an unsuspecting world, we'll be gone. And you might think this is wishful thinking, but it's much more than that. It's God-given conviction based on Bible truth and, in the following pages, you'll see what I mean.

> *"For the Lord Himself shall descend from Heaven with a shout, with the voice of the archangel, and with the trump of God: and the dead in Christ shall rise first; Then we who are alive and remain shall be caught up together with them in the clouds, to meet the Lord in the air: and so shall we ever be with the Lord."*
>
> ~ 1st Thessalonians 4:16-17

Chapter One

God's M.O.

M.O., OR MODUS OPERANDI, refers to a certain way of doing things. A way that's characteristic of the person in question. The phrase is often used by investigators when profiling suspects.

When there's a serial killer or rapist on the loose, the police will study that person's past crimes to see if there's a set pattern or certain method being used. For instance, is there a weapon of choice (gun vs knife)? Do all the victims have the same build, gender, ethnicity? Are they all from the same part of town? Did they all ride the bus, take the subway, drive a car? Were the crimes all committed the same time of day? By studying the past, the police observe common threads which help them predict when and where the suspect may strike again. And we can do the same. Not with suspects, but with God.

Wanna know what God's gonna do in the future? Then look to the Book and see what He's done in the past. The Lord has a certain way of doing things and, if there's one thing I know, He's very consistent.

- Before flooding the world, the Lord made sure that Noah and his family were safe in the ark.
- Before destroying Sodom and Gomorrah, the Lord made sure that Lot and his family had exited the cities.
- Before sending plagues on the land of Egypt, He first made sure that the children of Israel were safe in Goshen.
- Before drowning the Egyptians in the Red Sea, He first made sure that His people had made it across, that they were safely ashore on the other side.

I could continue, but I think you get the point. There's a definite pattern here, and the pattern is this: Before raining judgment down on the wicked, God rescues His own. And, if the past is any indication of the future (and it is), you can rest assured the Church will be gone before the tribulation hits.

Of course, some would argue that, since God didn't rescue Christians from being fed to the lions in Rome, and didn't rescue the Apostle Paul from being executed at the hands of Nero, the aforesaid conclusion is null-n-void. But is it? No, not really.

God had nothing to do with the persecution of Christians, and had nothing to do with Paul's execution. Whereas the worldwide flood, the destruction of Sodom and Gomorrah, and the Egyptian plagues were all caused by God. God *Himself* was the instigator and mastermind behind these things. And so the verdict stands: God rescues His own before *He Himself* rains judgment down on the wicked.

CHAPTER TWO

World Conditions

IMMEDIATLEY BEFORE THE RAPTURE there'll be buying and selling, eating and drinking, marrying and giving in marriage (Luke 17:28-30). In other words, it'll be business as usual. However, right before the second coming, it'll be anything but.

The second coming of Christ comes on the heels of the great tribulation and, during that time, the world will be decimated. There'll be famines and earthquakes, fatal diseases, riots, wars, mass starvation, wide-spread panic. An asteroid will hit the planet, all sea life will be wiped out, over half the Earth's population will be destroyed, and most who remain will beg to die.

By no stretch of the imagination can this be construed as the norm or *"business as usual."* But it's the plight of the world and the way things will be when Christ returns at the second coming.

Chapter Three

Restrainer Removed

THE BIBLE SAYS the Antichrist can't be revealed until the restrainer is removed (2nd Thessalonians 2:7-8). And, though some question whether the restrainer is the Holy Spirit or the Church, I believe it's both. It's the Holy Spirit operating through the Church.

Jesus said that we, as Believers, are the salt of the Earth and the light of the world. So it stands to reason that, when all the Believers suddenly vanish, the world will be plunged into darkness, i.e., civil unrest, anarchy, mob violence, and utter debauchery. Add to the mix economic collapse and you have all the ingredients for revolution. Like Germany in 1933, the world will be looking for a man. A man with a plan. For someone who'll step up to the plate and solve all their problems.

When all this happens, when these things start taking place and converge, the stage will be set and the players ready. Ready for Act Two, Scene One. And, in case you're wondering, Act One is the rapture. With the Church removed, the Antichrist will be free to move about at will. Free to abrogate laws, to usurp power, and free to execute his demonic scheme.

Chapter Four

The Seven Feasts

MORE THAN 1,400 YEARS before Christ was born, God gave seven Feasts to the nation of Israel. Seven Feasts commemorating past events and providing an outline of things to come. Leviticus 23 gives the annual order in which these Feasts are to be observed and, believe it or not, the fulfillment of these Feasts occur in that EXACT SAME ORDER. What's more, each occurs DURING THE ACTUAL FEAST, the Feast in question (the Feast depicting that event). It's like they've synchronized their watches!

It's no coincidence Christ was crucified during *the Feast of Passover.* It's no coincidence He rose from the dead during *the Feast of First Fruits.* It's no coincidence the Holy Spirit descended on Believers during *the Feast of Pentecost.** And it'll be no coincidence when Christians go flying through the air during *the Feast of Trumpets.* That's why, every September, I look to the skies with anticipation.

* As you can see, the Spring Feasts have already been fulfilled, and, in the very near future, the Fall Feasts will follow suit.

The next Feast, the one that follows *the Feast of Trumpets* (Yom Kippur), depicts the second coming of Christ, which clearly indicates the rapture comes first, *before* the second coming.

The seventh Feast, *the Feast of Tabernacles,* depicts Christ's millennial reign here on Earth when He "tabernacles" among His people.

Chapter Five

The Church Not Mentioned

THE BOOK OF REVELATION was written in chronological order and it's between chapters 5 and 20 that the tribulation takes place. What's conspicuous is that nowhere in these chapters is the Church ever mentioned. Though mentioned 19 times in the first three chapters, you won't find it anywhere in the next 16. Yes, the book alludes to the Church in chapter 19, calling her the bride of Christ. But that passage deals with events taking place in Heaven and not what's happening here on Earth.

Chapter Six

The Mark Not Mentioned

WHY WEREN'T THEY WARNED? Between Peter, Paul, James, John, and Jude, 21 letters were written to the early Church, yet nowhere in these letters is the *Mark of the Beast* mentioned, not even once. Which would seem really strange if these Believers were at risk. But the fact is, they weren't at risk. They weren't and they aren't.

Believers have never been at risk when it comes to the *Mark of the Beast*. As Christians, we'll be long gone before the Antichrist comes to power and before the mark is given. The only place you'll find the *Mark of the Beast* recorded in Scripture is in Revelation, after the Church has vanished.

The *Mark of the Beast* is the mark placed in the right hand or forehead during the tribulation. By receiving this mark, people will show their allegiance to the Antichrist, and will be allowed to buy and sell.

Though translated as 666 in English, we have no idea what language will be used, nor do we know if it will be an outward mark or an embedded chip. What we do know is that those receiving the mark will seal their fate. Once received, there's no turning back. See Revelation 13:16-18 and 14:9-11.

Chapter Seven

Jewish Wedding Customs

THE CHURCH IS THE BRIDE OF CHRIST, and, according to Jewish wedding customs, the groom returns home after proposing marriage. The groom returns home and his beloved bride remains behind. She remains at her parents' house until the wedding. And it's during this time, this time of separation, she prepares her bridal trousseau while the groom stays busy constructing the bridal chamber.

Jesus said, "*. . . I go to prepare a place for you. And if I go and prepare a place for you, I will come again and receive you unto myself; that where I am, there ye may be also*" (John 14:2-3).

When the time is right, the groom returns to fetch his bride and take her home. Home to his father's house where the marriage feast begins and continues for seven days.

We know from the book of Daniel that a day equals one year in Bible prophecy, and one week equals seven years. With this being the case, it's easy to connect the dots and conclude that the seven "days" of feasting coincide with the seven years of tribulation. And, if the two coincide, that puts the rapture at the very beginning of those seven years.

CHAPTER EIGHT

No Protection = Absence

IN REVELATION 7:3-4, we read where the Lord gives a special seal of protection to the 144,000 servants chosen from Israel. Then, later, in Revelation 9, we see this seal in action. We see it shielding from plagues, warding off scorpions, and protecting the 144,000. Which is great if you happen to be one of 'em.

But what about the Church? What about His blushing bride? Why would the Lord protect the 144,000 and not protect His own bride? The answer: He wouldn't. He wouldn't protect one without protecting the other, not if "*the other*" was still here. But the fact is, we won't be. We won't be here. At that point in time, the Church will have already left. We will have already split, vanished, vamoosed, flown the coop, skedaddled.

Chapter Nine

The 24 Elders

"Four and twenty elders fall down before Him that sat on the throne . . . and cast their crowns before the throne, saying, Thou art worthy, O Lord, to receive glory and honor and power . . ." (Revelation 4:10-11).

The 24 elders can't cast their crowns before they're given any more than a quarterback can pass the ball before it's snapped. You can't cast or pass something ya don't have, and the fact that the 24 elders already have their crowns in Revelation 4 means that, at that point in time, the Bema Seat of Christ has already happened.

The Bema Seat of Christ is where crowns are awarded, and if the Bema Seat has already happened by Revelation 4, so has the rapture. As mentioned, the book of Revelation was written in chronological order and, knowing the aforesaid events have all happened by chapter 4, and knowing the tribulation doesn't start till chapter 6, points to the obvious. Before the Antichrist takes over, before all hell breaks loose, the Church will be gone. As sure as day follows night, the casting of crowns follows the Bema Seat, and the Bema Seat follows the rapture (Romans 14:10; 1st Corinthians 3:12-15; and 2nd Corinthians 5:10).

Chapter Ten

Saved from Wrath

CHRISTIANS HAVE ALWAYS SUFFERED PERSECUTION. From being beaten and scourged to burned at the stake, our trials have been many. So why would the great tribulation be any different? What makes us think *we* can escape when so many haven't? That's a good question, and here's the answer: The great tribulation will be initiated by Christ, whereas Satan is the culprit behind all the other. See Revelation 5:9 and 16:1.

For centuries, Satan has tempted and tortured God's people, but that's about to end. His days are numbered. God is saying enough is enough and, like a mighty volcano, He's about to erupt. Exactly when this will happen, no one knows. But we know it'll happen and soon.

With all His fury, God will unleash His wrath on a wicked world, but the Christians will be gone. Wrath means fierce anger, and, since God isn't angry at Christians, there's no need for us to stick around. According to Scripture, Christians are saved from God's wrath, from ALL of God's wrath (Romans 5:9 and 1st Thessalonians 5:9), including the great tribulation. Which the Bible calls, *"THE GREAT DAY OF HIS WRATH . . ."* (Revelation 6:17).

Believe me, I've done plenty to provoke God's anger. But God redirected that anger toward Christ as He hung on the cross. And what He did for me, He did for you. God sent His Son to die in our place, to bear the punishment we deserve so we won't have to. But, as wonderful as this is, it's all for naught unless you accept it. Accept it by faith.

Christ is coming and coming soon.
And we'd best be ready. But how?

Keep reading . . . .

Chapter Eleven

Two Big Surprises

WE'LL HAVE TWO BIG SURPRISES when we get to Heaven. First, we'll be surprised at all those who made it. There'll be thieves and hookers and dopers in Heaven. That is, ex-thieves, ex-hookers, and ex-dopers. The second surprise? We'll be surprised at those we thought for sure would be there but aren't. Many church members, clerics, and upstanding members of the community will be noticeably absent.

The reason? Those we consider to be good moral people tend to rely on those things (on their perceived goodness and morality), whereas the moral degenerate and social outcast are keenly aware of their sin, and it's that awareness that drives them to their knees, that causes them to cry out to God for mercy. You'll see this illustrated in Luke 18:10-14.

According to Scripture, the plan of salvation is simple, and it's that simplicity that causes many to stumble. Becoming a Christian is easy and, in the minds of many, it's too easy. So, to raise the bar and make things more difficult, they've added some things. They've added requirements. Requirements the Lord never intended. In the following pages, we'll examine these things and see how Satan has muddied the water.

Chapter Twelve

Gift vs Reward

RECENTLY, WHILE VISITING A DOCTOR'S OFFICE, I overheard a little girl ask her grandma, *"Grandma, are you going to get me something for my birthday?"* and was shocked by Grandma's reply. Her grandma said, *"Well, now that depends . . . . Have you been a good little girl this year?"* Since when does a gift have strings attached? A gift by definition is FREE, and if ya gotta be good to get it, it's not a gift anymore. It's a REWARD!

Unfortunately, Grandma's logic isn't uncommon. It's a widespread misnomer, and no wonder. Every year at Christmastime, we brainwash the children with songs like *Santa Claus is Coming to Town.* Have you ever listened to the words of that song? In essence, it's saying that only good little boys and girls get gifts under the tree, and that bad boys and girls get absolutely nothing! I am soooooooo glad I didn't have to be a *"good little boy"* to receive God's gift of salvation. If being good was required, I'd be in a heap of trouble, and so would you.

> *"There is none that doeth good, no, not one"* (Psalms 14:3).
>
> *". . . There is none good but God"* (Mark 10:18).
>
> *"All we like sheep have gone astray . . ."* (Isaiah 53:6).
>
> *"For all have sinned . . ."* (Romans 3:23).
>
> *"The wages of sin is death, but the GIFT of God is eternal life through Jesus Christ, our Lord"* (Romans 6:23).

The wage is what we've earned, but the gift is freely given. Jesus collected our wages by dying on the cross. It was His precious blood that paid the price and purchased this gift. And now it's ours for the asking. *"For whosoever shall call upon the name of the Lord shall be saved"* (Romans 10:13). That's right, whosoever. That means that no matter who you are or what you've done, God still loves you and wants to forgive.

Salvation may be free, but it's not cheap. It cost God His only Son, and cost Jesus His life's blood.

Chapter Thirteen

Hard vs Easy

WHAT'S THE DIFFERENCE between hard and easy, and what's considered hard? What about flying through the air without any props or planes? Would that be hard? Well, it really depends on who you're asking. For Betty the Bird or Barney the Bumble Bee, such a feat would be easy. But for the rest of us, and for Larry the Caterpillar, we're pretty much grounded.

However, unlike the rest of us, Larry will eventually fly. Larry the Caterpillar will eventually soar through the air, fly through the breeze, and flutter to his heart's content. And no, he won't go to flight school, won't join the Air Force, and won't study aeronautics. But what this grubby little creature will do is experience the miracle we call metamorphosis. One day Larry will spin a cocoon around himself and, soon thereafter, will emerge as a beautyful butterfly. Then, on that very day, Larry will fly! What once was impossible will then become possible. And not only possible, but easy.

What about keeping God's law? Is that hard or easy? It really depends on who you're asking. For the Spirit-filled Christian, such a feat would be easy. But for the unregenerate, for those who don't know the Lord, keeping God's law is extremely difficult, if not impossible. And how could it not be?

We're all born with a sin nature, a natural bent toward evil, and it's only through the second birth that anyone receives a new nature. The Bible says our hearts are "*. . . deceitful above all things and desperately wicked . . .*" (Jeremiah 17:9) but, through the miracle of the second birth, God performs surgery. Heart surgery. He performs a spiritual heart transplant, giving us a new heart. A new heart with new hopes, new thoughts, and new desires. See Ezekiel 36:26-27.

We're given a whole new outlook. An outlook with divine perspective. We start seeing things through God's eyes, the way He sees them. "*If any man be in Christ,*" the Bible says, "*he is a new creation; old things have passed away and, behold, all things have become new*" (2nd Corinthians 5:17). As with Larry the Caterpillar, once we've experienced the second birth, the impossible becomes possible. And not only possible, but easy.

That's why salvation *must* come first. Before baptism, catechism, discipleship, or adhering to any rules, we must first be saved. An unsaved person has neither the desire nor ability to obey God but, the moment we're saved, the moment we receive Christ, everything changes. The Holy Spirit takes up residence inside of us and goes to work. The Bible says, *"God is at work within you both to will and to do of His good pleasure"* (Philippians 2:13).

Keep in mind this promise is for the Believer and not the lost. It doesn't apply to the unbeliever. If you're not a born again Christian, the Spirit of God doesn't live in you. He *wants* to live in you, and will if you'll let Him. But it's up to you. *"Believe on the Lord Jesus Christ and thou shalt be saved . . ."* (Acts 16:31).

Once inside the new Believer, God imparts His love (Romans 5:5). And it's this love that constrains us (2nd Corinthians 5:14). That drives, compels, and motivates. If I tried keeping God's law in the past, before becoming a Christian, it was done out of fear. Fear of divine judgment. But now that I'm saved and filled with God's love, it's a whole new ballgame. There's new motivation.

Nowadays when keeping God's law (refraining from murder, theft, lies, adultery, etc.), it's because I care. I care for the would-be victims. I don't wanna hurt 'em. In fact, instead of hurting them, I'm wanting to help. Despite my self-centered past, I find myself pitching in, getting involved, and wanting to help. This is what the Scripture means when it says, "*Love is the fulfillment of the law*" (Romans 13:10).

Once you're filled with God's love, you catch yourself keeping God's law. Like breathing in and out, it becomes automatic. Thus saith the Lord, "*I will put my Spirit within you, and cause you to walk in my statutes, and ye shall keep mine ordinances and do them*" (Ezekiel 36:27).

So does this mean God forces obedience? No, not really. No more than He forces the fish to swim or the birds to fly. He gives us the desire and ability, but no one is forced.

There's a natural flow to all this. First, we hear the Gospel message. Second, we place our faith in Christ, receiving Him as Savior. Third, the Lord enters our bodies, indwelling us by His Holy Spirit. Fourth, we surrender ourselves to the lordship of Christ, and fifth, the Spirit fills us with God's love. Then, soon thereafter, we start showing this love to others.

In writing to the Church, to born again Christians, Paul instructs us to be filled with the Spirit (Ephesians 5:18). And yes, as Christians, we already have the Holy Spirit, having received Him at the time of conversion (Romans 8:9), which is a one-time experience. But being filled with the Spirit is different and happens repeatedly (or should happen repeatedly), again and again throughout our Christian walk. Our gas tanks need refilling from time to time, and so do we.

For more on this, see Billy Graham's book entitled *The Holy Spirit: Activating God's Power in Your Life.*

Having committed adultery, King David worried that God might take the Holy Spirit from him (Psalm 51:11). So why didn't the Corinthian Christians committing fornication worry about the same?

The answer to this shows a stark contrast and exemplifies the difference between the old and new covenants, or one of the differences. When David committed adultery, Christ had not yet died. Which means payment for David's sin hadn't been made, and wouldn't be made for another 1,000 years. Whereas the sins committed in Corinth were committed after the cross. After the cross and after the resurrection.

As New Testament Believers, we enjoy a promise that was never given to Old Testament saints: Thus saith the Lord, "*. . . I will never leave thee, nor forsake thee*" (Hebrews 13:5). If you're a born again Christian, the Lord is with you *always* via the Holy Spirit.

Chapter Fourteen

Messy House

I HATE TO ADMIT IT, BUT I'm not the world's best housekeeper. In fact, my place makes Oscar Madison look good. So when I saw this maid service advertised in Sunday's paper, it got my attention. Suppose I arranged for one of their maids to clean my house next Saturday at 10 a.m. Only problem is there are five whole days between now and then. That's five whole days in which to forget. And no, I'm not likely to forget. But pretend I do.

Saturday morning finally arrives and, at 10 a.m., the doorbell rings. Setting my bowl of Cheerios down on the counter, I go to the door, look through the peephole and, sure enough, it's the maid. Yup, it's the maid. IT'S THE MAID!!! Shocked and panicked, I spring into action. *"Just a minute!"* I shout as I start picking up, frantically rushing through the house, running from room to room, trying to make a dent, trying to make a difference.

I'm picking up clothes, cramming things in the closet, shoving papers under the bed when, once again, the doorbell rings. But this time I answer. I go to the front, open the door and, with the sincerest apology I can possibly muster, I say, "*I am so sorry, Maria, but the place is a mess. Is there any way you could come back tomorrow? If you come back tomorrow, I promise to have things in order. The dishes will be washed, the floors swept, and the furniture polished. I just need more time. Can you please give me more time?*"

I hope you know this is just an illustration. I'm not really that dumb. Had I actually made such a request, Maria would have thought me loco, i.e., a few bricks shy of a load, a few fries short of a Happy Meal, a few . . . . Okay, well, you know. She would have answered, "*Kind sir, you don't understand. That's **MY** job. That's why **I'M** here. That's what **I** do.*"

Jesus said, *"Behold, I stand at the door and knock; if anyone hears my voice and opens the door, I will come in . . ."* Our Lord entreats men and women with His love, wooing them with compassion, knocking on their heart's door. But, all too often, the reply He gets is, *"I'm so sorry, Lord, but my life is a mess. I just need more time — time to get my act together."* What they fail to realize is that that's **His** job. That's why **He's** here. That's what **He** does.

Our Lord specializes in cleaning up lives and mending broken people. Stop trying to do it on your own and come to the Lord just as you are. With all of your hurts, all of your faults, and all of your problems. He loves you with all His heart and waits with open arms.

CHAPTER FIFTEEN

What About Repentance?

JESUS SAID, *"Except ye repent, ye shall all likewise perish."* So when someone asks if repentance is required for salvation, my answer is an emphatic *yes!* Repentance *IS* required, but not the repentance that most folks think of when they hear the word. Over the years, the meaning has changed. In the mind of the public, repent and repentance don't mean what they used to.

We've seen it before, how definitions change with the passing of time. When words are misused (used in the wrong context) by a large number of people, and that misuse continues over a period of time, such words take on a whole new meaning. The original meaning is greatly obscured and sometimes obliterated.

Take the word *gay* for instance. Thirty years ago we'd talk about *gay Paree,* but nowadays it's *gay San Francisco,* and one has nothing to do with the other. The meaning has changed. The word has been totally revised and its new definition has no resemblance to the old. It doesn't mean what it used to.

The word *conversation* is another example. The Apostle Paul wrote to the early church saying, "*Let your conversation be without covetousness . . .*" (Hebrews 13:5). But this quote is taken from an Old English Bible and, in 1611, when that Bible was first published, *conversation* meant something entirely different. Back then it meant conduct or behavior, whereas today it means a verbal dialog between two or more people. The word has changed, and its new definition is totally different from the old. It doesn't mean what it used to.

The Greek word for *repent* is metanoēte, and, simply put, means to change one's mind. This happens the moment we're saved. We change our minds from one of unbelief to belief. But this definition is totally foreign to most folks. In the mind of the public, the vast majority of the English-speaking world, the word *repent* means to stop sinning. And to suggest that someone must stop sinning to be saved is nothing less than heresy.

One of the main purposes of *The Gospel According to John* is to win the lost (John 20:31). Yet not even once does the word *repent* appear in that Gospel. You won't find it there. Nor will you find it in Acts 16.

And, speaking of Acts 16, it's very significant what the Apostle Paul said to the Philippian jailer when asked, *"What must I do to be saved?"* Paul answered, *"Believe on the Lord Jesus Christ and thou shalt be saved . . ."* (Acts 16:31). But what's just as significant is what Paul didn't say. Nowhere in this passage is the word *repent* ever mentioned, which begs the question: If repentance is required for salvation, why didn't Paul say so? Why didn't John say so? Why isn't it mentioned??

Repentance isn't mentioned in these passages because doing so would be redundant. If you're told to believe and, up till that moment, have never known anything but unbelief, then changing your mind is the only way you can possibly start believing. It goes without saying, which is often the case.

Example: I could say, "*The ship was lost beneath the cold frozen ice,*" but two of those words aren't needed. I mean, ice isn't ICE unless it's frozen, and have you ever known ice NOT to be cold? Some things are automatically understood and don't need to be mentioned.

But the redundancy thing isn't why I won't use the word *repent* anymore. I avoid that word like the plague because of its new definition. As stated, the vast majority of the English-speaking world thinks that *repent* means to stop sinning.

To the woman caught in adultery, Jesus said, *"Neither do I condemn thee: Go, and sin no more"* (John 8:11). And yes, she was told to *"sin no more,"* but note the sequence. It wasn't till AFTER she had already been forgiven! The forgiveness wasn't contingent upon her ability to abstain. The Lord didn't say, *"I won't condemn you IF you'll promise to sin no more."* Had that been the case, had our Lord said such a thing, her salvation would have been a reward for her works and not a gift of grace. And, had that been the case, God's word would then be a lie, for the Scripture says, *"By grace are ye saved through faith; and not of yourselves, it is the GIFT of God. Not of works, lest any man should boast"* (Ephesians 2:8-9).

> There's a big difference between changing your mind and changing your behavior. Before you'll ever experience any significant change in behavior, you must first experience a change of heart. And we can no more change our wicked hearts than a tiny baby can change its dirty diaper. Babies need their parents, and we need the Lord.

Many say you must "*turn from sin*" in order to be saved, which is just another way of saying that you gotta stop sinning to be saved, which is nothing but malarkey, a bunch of malarkey. It's another version of salvation by works, and if you don't think abstaining from sin is work, just ask someone with an addiction. Resisting drugs, overcoming alcohol, or abstaining from illicit sex is no easy task. Not when everything within you craves satisfaction and is screaming for relief. Apart from God's indwelling presence, giving up those things is extremely difficult. And if that's not *work,* I don't know what is.

Some concede that you don't need to stop sinning to be saved but quickly add, "*Yeah, but . . .*" Not willing to accept God's gift as a gift, with no strings attached, they say, "*Yeah, but ya gotta be WILLING to stop sinning.*"

When my parents presented me with a brand new bicycle on my 10th birthday, all they said was, "*Happy Birthday!*" But suppose they had said something else. Suppose they had said, "*Son, we're thinking about giving you this new bike but, before we do, you must first tell us that you're willing to stop popping your knuckles.*" Had that been the case, had my parents said such a thing, that bike would not have been a gift. It may have been a bribe, and it may have been an incentive, but it would not have been a gift. Not if strings were attached. A gift isn't a gift unless it's FREE.

> "*. . . The GIFT of God is eternal life through Jesus Christ, our Lord*" (Romans 6:23).

Don't get me wrong. I'm not saying we should continue in sin. I'm just saying that giving up sin isn't a condition for salvation. It's not a prerequisite. But, once saved, we should definitely stop sinning. Or at least make the effort. As children of God, we should resist every temptation and serve the Lord with all our hearts.

With that said, I should quickly add that we will never be sinless. Not in this life. As we grow in Christ, we will sin less and less, but will never be sinless. Not as long as we remain in these mortal bodies (Ecclesiastes 7:20). That's why we'll always need God's mercy, and why the blood of Christ is *continually* cleansing us from every sin (1st John 1:7).

Yes, the Scripture says, "*Whosoever is born of God doth not commit sin . . .*" (1st John 3:9), but the word *commit* (as used here) is best rendered practice. Simply put, once you're born again, you won't habitually practice sin as a way of life. But that doesn't mean you won't ever sin again. Show me someone who thinks they've achieved sinless perfection, and I'll show you a modern day Pharisee, someone who's semi-conceited and filled with pride.

In contrast, there's the person who says they're a Christian but lives like the devil. Chances are that person has never been saved. They may have been baptized, and may have joined the church, but anyone who habitually sins has never been saved or born again.

The Old Testament Hebrew words for "repent" are nacham and shuwb. And no, there's no hidden meaning. Unlike their New Testament counterpart, these words mean exactly what's commonly believed. Nacham means to have regret, and shuwb means to turn or return. But here's the danger: Taking a New Testament Greek word and trying to squeeze it into an Old Testament Hebrew definition is like trying to force a square peg into a round hole. It won't fit.

Chapter Sixteen

Two Natures

THOUGH GIVEN A NEW NATURE AT CONVERSION, we still have the old. Yup, that's right. Christians have two natures. Two natures that are diametrically opposed (Galatians 5:17). It's like there's a Dr. Jekyll and Mr. Hyde living in each of us. But, unlike the story, our Dr. Jekyll isn't subject to Mr. Hyde, which is to say that our new nature isn't subject to the old. The Lord gives us an escape out of every temptation (1st Corinthians 10:13) and so, when we sin, there's no excuse. We can't say, *"I couldn't help myself"* because we could. We could and we can.

Our so-called excuses won't fly. Thank God we're justified by the blood of Christ and not our excuses (Romans 5:9).

So, potentially, Christians can resist every temptation, but the reality is we don't. Consider Romans 7:15-18 where Paul explains, "*For what I am doing, I don't understand; for I am not practicing the things I would like to do, but am doing the very things I hate. And, if I hate the things I'm doing, I agree with the Law, that it is good. So now, it is no longer I that am doing it, but sin that dwelleth in me. For I know that nothing good is in me, that is, in my flesh; for the willingness is present, but the doing of the good is not.*"

Perhaps Jesus said it best. "*. . . truly the spirit is willing, but the flesh is weak*" (Mark 14:38). However, before taking this as a license to sin, you might wanna check the context: "*Watch and pray, lest ye enter into temptation; truly the spirit is willing, but the flesh is weak.*" So no, there's no license here, but an admonition to spend more time in prayer.

Of course, communication with God is a two-way street. We speak to Him through prayer, and He speaks to us through His word, the Holy Bible. His word is our spiritual sustenance (Matthew 4:4), the key to spiritual growth (1st Peter 2:2), and insulation against sin. The psalmist prayed, *"Thy word have I hid in mine heart, that I might not sin against thee"* (Psalm 119:11).

When tempted by Satan, Jesus responded to each temptation by quoting Scripture, and we should do the same. But ya can't quote it if ya don't know it. So spending time in God's word becomes priority.

> Two passions beat within my chest. One is foul and the other blessed. The one I love and the other I hate. But the one I feed will dominate.

CHAPTER SEVENTEEN

What it Means to Believe

JOHN 3:16 IS CRYSTAL CLEAR, yet some try to confuse things by redefining believe. Exactly what does it mean to believe? Okay, I admit the Greek word for *believe* (pisteuo) can be translated as *commit.* But here's the danger: The English word *commit* has at least ten definitions, and only one of 'em fits. Pick the wrong definition and you'll end up trusting in works, i.e., salvation by dedication as opposed to grace.

Most folks think of commitment in terms of relationships and, usually, in terms of marriage. When a bride and groom stand before the preacher to exchange vows, they're committing themselves to each other *"till death do we part."* And many surmise this is what's needed for salvation. They think we must promise or commit ourselves to serve the Lord for the rest of our days. Such a commitment is great and highly commendable, but not if used as a bargaining chip.

If a person surrenders their life to the Lord in hopes that the Lord will return the favor by saving their soul, that person is missing the whole concept of grace. Such logic is nothing more than bartering, and bartering with an IOU. It's man trying to buy his own salvation on credit, i.e., buy now, pay later.

They think they can receive the Lord's forgiveness today with no money down, then pay Him back later with a lifetime of service. What they fail to realize is that salvation is FREE. It's a GIFT and not a loan! You will never ever have to repay Him because the price has already been paid! If you want to serve the Lord, that's great. But know this: The Lord will save you by His grace whether you ever serve Him or not.

The ones trying to repay God for salvation are easy to spot. They're the ones who think they can lose it. They're busy making their monthly payments to the Lord in the form of good deeds, and they carry this awful fear. They fear that, should they ever miss a few payments (backslide and sin), the Lord will send forth Guido and repossess their salvation.

Question: Why do bankers repossess cars?

Answer: Because of nonpayment.

Question: Why will the Lord never repossess our salvation?

Answer: Because the full payment has already been made. Salvation was never bought on credit, but was paid for in advance by the blood of Jesus.

So if the Greek word for believe and commit doesn't mean surrendering ourselves in servitude, what does it mean? To answer this question, I'd like to talk Tarzan.

Some vines are stronger than others, which is a major concern if you're going to be swinging from tree to tree. In this story, YOU are the new Tarzan, and today is your first day on the job. The assignment: You're to climb that tree over there, grab the vine, and jump! Sounds simple, doesn't it? Only problem is a) The spot you'll be jumping from is 40 feet off the ground; b) you failed to renew your Weight Watchers membership; and c) you're really not too sure about this vine. I mean . . . . will it hold?

Of course, this whole scenario is a metaphor. The tree represents all your perceived goodness and good deeds. The vine represents God's grace and mercy. And your body? Your body represents you, your eternal spirit. Committing the entire weight of your body to the vine is like committing yourself to God's saving grace.

As you can readily see, the word *commit,* as used here, means *to entrust something to another* or *to rely on.* Like throwing ourselves on the mercy of the court, we cast ourselves onto God's grace and mercy (the vine), entrusting Him with our eternal spirit. And, as we do, we stop relying on ourselves. We stop relying on our own perceived goodness (the tree) and start relying on the vine, God's amazing grace.

The Random House Dictionary gives many definitions for commit, but the one I've been looking for, the only one that fits in regards to salvation, is this: "*To entrust something to another, especially for safekeeping.*"

Believe it or not, everyone commits. We commit something to someone every day of the week. We commit our money to the bank, our gas to the tank, and the yard work to Frank. As responsible drivers, we commit our cars to mechanics, entrusting them with the maintenance and repair. As busy parents, we commit our children to daycares, entrusting them with their oversight and protection. As guilty sinners, we commit ourselves to the Savior, entrusting Him with our forgiveness and salvation. The only difference is that the mechanics and daycares (and Frank) will be sending us a bill, whereas Jesus offers His service at no cost.

> Though mercy and grace are closely related, they're not the same. God shows mercy by withholding all the terrible judgment we deserve, and shows grace by giving us all the wonderful blessings we don't deserve. He can do this because of what Jesus did at the cross. Jesus took all of our judgment so we can now enjoy all of His blessings.

Chapter Eighteen

Lifetime Commitment?

See Chapter Seventeen.

Chapter Nineteen

Public Profession of Faith?

CAN A PERSON BE SAVED in the privacy of their own home when there's no one around, or is a public profession of faith required? The answer is yes and no. Yes, you can be saved when there's no one around, and no, a public profession of faith is not required. Not to be saved, not to become a child of God. But to be an *obedient* child of God, once you're saved, you'll want to make it public. This can be done by walking the aisle during an altar call, and is definitely done when baptized. But no, a public profession of faith is not required for salvation.

True, Jesus said, "*Whosoever confesses me before men, him will I also confess before my Father in Heaven,*" but this is done *after* conversion and not before. Out of the abundance of the heart, the mouth speaketh. Once the Lord fills your heart, you won't be able to keep quiet. You'll want to shout it from the mountaintops and tell the whole world. "*Whosoever believeth on Him shall not be ashamed*" (Romans 10:11).

Billy Graham would often say, *"Everyone Jesus called in the New Testament, He called publicly."* But is that true? Our Lord was alone with Nicodemus in John, chapter 3, and alone with the Samaritan woman in John, chapter 4, when each was offered the gift of salvation.

Chapter Twenty

Give Your Life to Christ?

ASKING FOLKS TO GIVE THEIR LIVES TO CHRIST is a good thing, but only if those folks are already Christians. Asking a lost person to give their life to Christ is like asking them to trade, or that's how it's taken. If an unbeliever is asked to give anything to Christ (whether it's their heart, their life, or stamp collection), it constitutes a trade. Their thing in exchange for His thing, i.e., eternal life. And that, my friend, is just another form of salvation by works. It's man trying to purchase what God has freely given. See Romans 6:23 and Ephesians 2:8.

Generally speaking, once we receive this wonderful gift, once we've experienced the Lord's forgiveness, we *want* to give Him our lives. But not in order to get something. Rather, we give Him our lives as an expression of gratitude for what we already got. "*This is love, not that we loved God, but that He loved us . . . We love Him because He first loved us*" (1st John 4:10 and 19).

Instead of coercing unbelievers to give their lives to Christ, we should be telling them about the One who gave His life for them.

The Apostle Paul gives this mandate: "*I beseech you therefore, brethren, by the mercies of God, that you present your bodies as a living sacrifice . . .*" (Romans 12:1). But notice that Paul isn't saying this to the unbeliever. He's saying this to Christians, to the born again child of God. So yes, sacrifice and surrender *are* required of Christians, but Christians only. Quoting Romans 12:1 to an unbeliever is like having them read someone else's mail.

Bottom Line: Salvation has absolutely nothing to do with what we've done (or will do) for God, but has *everything* to do with what God did for us. He sent His only Son to die in our place, to bear the punishment we deserve so we won't have to. Christ died for our sins, rose again, and now offers forgiveness to everyone everywhere. Forgiveness and eternal life.

Getting saved is just a matter of receiving a gift, and how hard can that be? It shouldn't be hard at all and isn't, unless you're filled with pride. Pride keeps a person from acknowledging their sin and need of forgiveness.

If you don't think you're all that bad, why would Jesus die for your sins? If all we were guilty of were minor offenses, the Lord could have taken a slap on the wrist for our sins. He could have paid a really small fine. But that's not what He did. Christ *died* for our sins, and the mere fact that He went to such an extreme as to *die* for our sins means that we're guilty of sins deserving of death.

Compared with family and friends, you may not seem that bad. You may not seem bad at all. But compared to a holy God, you don't measure up. None of us do. That's why we need salvation. We're all guilty sinners in need of the Savior (Romans 3:23).

CHAPTER TWENTY-ONE

Make Jesus Lord?

THE QUESTION IS OFTEN ASKED, *"Have you made Jesus the Lord of your life?"* Which is like asking someone if they've made the sky blue. You can't make the sky blue because it's already blue. The sky's already blue and Jesus is already the Lord of your life. He's Lord of *everyone's* life. See Acts 10:36 and Romans 10:12.

But, in all fairness, I think we know what they're really asking. They're asking if we've surrendered ourselves to the lordship of Christ. And, without question, everyone should surrender to the lordship of Christ. But what I'd like to ask is this: Is such a surrender required for salvation? Is that a prerequisite? Because of Romans 10:9, most evangelicals would say yes. But, unfortunately, that verse has been misconstrued. Take a look . . . .

"If thou shalt confess with thy mouth the Lord Jesus, and shalt believe in thine heart that God hath raised him from the dead, thou shalt be saved."

To confess simply means *to acknowledge* or *agree with.* So confessing Jesus as Lord is simply acknowledging the fact that He *is* Lord. However, acknowledging His lordship and surrendering to His lordship are two different things. Yes, a person can be a born again Christian without having surrendered to the lordship of Christ, which explains the Corinthian church (1st Corinthians 3:3 and 5:1).

The Corinthian church was steeped in carnality and, based on their conduct, you would have never known they were Christians. Based on their conduct, you couldn't tell any difference between them and the lost. Yet the Apostle Paul still called them brethren and said they were in Christ. Albeit they were *babes* in Christ, they were still in Christ. Clearly, the Corinthian Believers had not surrendered to the lordship of Christ, but they were Believers nonetheless. They were still born again and headed for Heaven.

Chapter Twenty-Two

Salvation vs Discipleship

EVANGELIST BENNY HINN once said, *"Salvation is a free gift, but it will cost you your life."* What I'd like to know is this: If it costs you anything, anything at all, how can it be free? It can't! Benny is making a dreadful mistake and, unfortunately, it's a fairly common mistake. He's confusing salvation with discipleship.

Yes, the disciples were first called Christians in Antioch. And Chevrolets were first called cars in Detroit. But that doesn't mean every car rolling off the assembly line is a Chevy, nor does it mean that every Christian is a disciple. The words are not synonymous. All true disciples of Christ are definitely Christians, but not all Christians are disciples, and here's why: Not all Christians are willing to pay the cost of discipleship. Jesus said, *"Whosoever does not bear his cross, and come after me, cannot be my disciple"* (Luke 14:27).

With that said, please know that the Christians who don't pay the cost of discipleship are still Christians. In other words, if they were to die tonight, they'd still go to Heaven. They may not have many rewards once they got there, but they'd still get there.

Denying yourself and taking up your cross is not a requirement for salvation. If it was, if we had to bear a cross to be saved, then salvation would no longer be a gift of God's grace but a reward for our works, which is *ludicrous* and flies in the face of everything Christ died for!!

> "*Not by works of righteousness which we have done, but according to his mercy he saved us . . .*" (Titus 3:5).

Jesus bore HIS CROSS for all of us and, when it comes to salvation, that's the *only cross* we will ever need. Yes, as Christians, we should answer the call to discipleship, but don't confuse discipleship with salvation, and don't be telling the unbeliever to *"take up your cross and follow Christ"* lest he think that that's what's needed to enter Heaven. First get 'em saved, and then challenge them with discipleship.

CHAPTER TWENTY-THREE

What About Baptism?

IF SALVATION IS BY GRACE THROUGH FAITH, how do you explain Acts 2:38? That's where the Apostle Peter says, "*Repent, and be baptized, every one of you, in the name of Jesus Christ, for the forgiveness of sins.*" This certainly sounds like we must first be baptized. So what gives? Is water baptism required or not? Consider the following:

- Thief on the Cross: The thief on the cross died having never been baptized, yet Jesus assured him saying, "*This day shalt thou be with me in paradise*" (Luke 23:43).

- Acts, Chapter 10: Note the sequence of events in this passage. Peter has been sent to preach the Gospel to a group of Gentiles and, as he's preaching, all who hear and believe get saved. This (the salvation experience) happens in verse 44, but it's not till verse 48 they're commanded to be baptized.

- Inerrancy of Scripture: Since the overall teaching of Scripture is that salvation is received by grace and grace alone, Acts 2:38 would be an apparent contradiction. Which is to say that it *seems* that way but isn't. The Bible is the infallible* word of God, and God never contradicts Himself. If you ever come across a verse of Scripture that seems contradictory to another verse of Scripture, rest assured it isn't. There's an explanation. There's *always* an explanation. You may have to dig to find it (spend some time in prayer and study), but seek and ye shall find.

* Though flaws and errors can be found in modern translations of the Bible, its original Greek and Hebrew manuscripts are infallible.

Peter's command to *"repent, and be baptized . . . for the forgiveness of sins . . ."* implies that forgiveness is contingent upon baptism. But this is clearly refuted in the Greek. The Greek command to repent is in the second person plural, whereas the command to be baptized is in the third person singular. This, combined with the fact that the pronoun *your* (in the phrase *"forgiveness of your sins"*) is also second person plural, shows an important distinction.

Changing from second person plural to third person singular, then back again, links the phrase *"forgiveness of your sins"* directly to the command to repent. In English, this change in person and plurality would best be rendered, *"You* (plural) *repent for the forgiveness of your* (plural) *sins, and let each one of you* (singular) *be baptized."* Or, to be more succinct: *"All of you repent for the forgiveness of all your sins, and let each one of you be baptized."*

So no, water baptism is not required. Not to be saved. However, once saved, you should definitely get baptized. Our Lord commands it and, if you're going to live a life that's pleasing to Him, you'll want to be baptized. Baptism symbolizes the death, burial, and resurrection of Christ. And, because it's done in public, you'll be showing the world that you belong to Him.

CHAPTER TWENTY-FOUR

False Hope

AT THE CLOSE OF THE BROADCAST, TV preachers often lead their viewers in a revised version of the sinner's prayer. Viewers are asked to repeat the prayer word for word and, usually, the prayer goes something like this: *"Lord Jesus, I repent of my sins. Come into my heart. I make you my Lord and Savior."* Which is all well and good, but . . . .

More often than not, the cross is never mentioned. More often than not, nothing is said about Christ's vicarious death or His bodily resurrection. Which means, more often than not, the prayer is totally useless. You can ask Jesus into your heart all day long but, until you realize (and believe) that He died for your sins and rose again, it ain't gonna happen.

Such prayers, prayed without an understanding of the Gospel, are an exercise in futility. And what's worse is the false hope. False hope, false assurance, and false security. Believe it or not, these prayers are inoculating folks against conviction. After praying such a prayer, the preacher often looks into the camera and says, *"Friend, if you prayed that simple prayer, we believe you got born again."* And, with this assurance, many viewers shrug off future conviction and step into eternity thinking they're saved.

On Judgment Day, many will say, *"Lord, Lord, have we not walked the aisle and joined the church? Have we not been baptized? Have we not given our lives to Christ and made Jesus Lord?"* Then, to their utter shock, the Lord will reply, *"Depart from me, ye workers of iniquity: I never knew you"* (Matthew 7:23).

I said it before and I'll say it again. Salvation has absolutely nothing to do with what we've done (or will do) for God, but has *everything* to do with what God did for us at the cross.

As a nine-year-old boy, I walked the aisle during an altar call and was told that Christ died for me. But I had also been told that every U.S. soldier who gave his life on a foreign battle field died for me. And, in my nine-year-old mind, I couldn't see the difference. If only someone had explained to me that Christ died FOR MY SINS (and rose again), I would have been saved much sooner.

Thank God that, at the age of 15, I finally realized He died for my sins, taking upon Himself all the punishment I deserve. Not to disparage our troops and all they have done to preserve our freedoms, none of 'em have died for my sins.

CHAPTER TWENTY-FIVE

Grace vs Law

WHETHER IT'S THE MOSAIC LAW or our own code of conduct, the Law (in the broadest sense) is any set of rules we try to follow in hopes that keeping those rules will earn God's favor and acceptance.

> **The Bad News**: As descendants of Adam, with a fallen nature, we can never be good enough to earn God's favor.
>
> **The Good News**: Since Jesus was born of a virgin, He didn't have the fallen nature and, through perfect obedience, fulfilled the Law. Hence, He was qualified to die in our place. Having no sin of His own, He went to the cross and died for ours.

So now, because of the cross, God's favor and acceptance are freely given. They're a gift of grace. And grace is unmerited favor. Unearned, undeserved, unmerited favor.

As born again Christians, we're no longer under the Law of Moses, but now adhere to the Law of Christ (Romans 6:14; Galatians 6:2; and 1st John 3:23). And they differ in many respects. But perhaps the most notable is purpose.

Through the indwelling presence of the Holy Spirit, God enables Christians to keep the Law of Christ. However, when the Mosaic Law was first given, He knew full well that neither Jew nor Gentile would ever be able to keep it. Not on their own. Not completely. So why bother? Why bother giving laws that no one can keep? There are three reasons:

#1 To set the standard;

#2 To make us realize we can never live up to that standard on our own; and

#3 To show us our need for mercy.

The Law of Moses and the Law of Christ also differ in sacrifice. The Law of Moses requires that bulls, sheep, and goats be sacrificed and sacrificed on a continuing basis, whereas the Law of Christ is satisfied by that one supreme sacrifice. The sacrifice He made at the cross. By dying on the cross, Christ made the full and final payment for all our sins, becoming the ultimate sacrifice for all mankind.

But, aside from differences, how are they alike? Do the two have anything in common? Jesus said, "*A new commandment I give unto you, that ye love one another.*" And, believe it or not, this new commandment is an abbreviation of the old. Paul explains: "*He that loveth another hath fulfilled the law*" (Romans 13:8).

In other words, if you really love someone, you won't be lying to them. If you really love someone, you won't be stealing from them. If you really love someone, you won't be trying to kill 'em, etc. If you really and truly love others the way the Lord loves you, you'll automatically be keeping the Law, both the Law of Christ and the moral aspects of the Mosaic Law.

But we can no more keep the Law of Christ than we kept the Law of Moses, not on our own. And we can never love others on our own, not the way we should. Jesus said, "*Without me ye can do nothing*" (John 15:5). That's why we *must* be born again and filled with the love that only He can give. See Romans 5:5 and Galatians 5:22.

The bloodline of man was contaminated by Adam's sin. Which means we've all inherited the sin nature. All of us but Jesus. As you know, Mary was a virgin. The baby Jesus was conceived by the Holy Spirit and not Joseph. Unlike the rest of us, Jesus was sinless at birth, and remained sinless throughout His life.

But what about Mary? Wasn't Mary a descendant of Adam? Hadn't she inherited the sin nature? And, of course, the answer is yes. So wouldn't she have passed that nature on to Jesus? And the answer is no. A baby's blood is derived from its father, not its mother. And, though mother and child are connected by the umbilical cord during gestation, the blood of one never passes to the other. Acting as a barrier, the placenta keeps the two from mingling.

> We're not sinners because we sin. Rather, we sin because we're sinners. We were born that way (Psalms 51:5). However, by being born again, we receive a new nature and can overcome sin's power.

CHAPTER TWENTY-SIX

Horrific Tragedy

JOHN GRIFFITH, ALONG WITH HIS WIFE and young son, settled near the Mississippi River where he found a job working as a switchman on a drawbridge. A fascinating job that impressed his son and garnered great respect. And oh how his son wanted to come. He wanted to be there. He wanted to tag along and see Dad in action. So Dad made a promise. He promised his boy that, as soon as the school year ended, he could come. He could join him on the job and they'd make a day of it.

Upon hearing these words, the boy jumped for joy. With cartwheels and backflips, he welcomed the news. But the wait would be arduous. As days turned to weeks, and weeks to months, time seemed to drag.

When the day finally arrived, the boy leaped into the truck at the crack of dawn and, riding shotgun, was beside himself with anticipation. Once on site, he beamed with pride watching Dad operate the controls. He watched as Dad raised and lowered the bridge. Again and again, he watched in awe, with wide-eyed amazement. Surely, he thought, *"Dad must be the greatest man alive. How can one man, single-handedly, control such a massive structure?"*

Before they knew it, it was noon and time to eat. John had just raised the bridge, allowing ships to pass. Then, taking their lunch pails, they walked to a nearby park and commenced to munch. As they ate, John told stories to his son. In vivid detail, he told about the enormous ships they were seeing and their marvelous destinations. He told story after story, with his boy hanging on every word. Lost in a world of wonder, the boy imagined all the exotic places and how thrilling it'd be to sail the seven seas. But their midday meal was abruptly ended by the shrieking sound of a distant train whistle.

Looking at his watch, John was alarmed to see that it was already 1:07. The bridge was still raised and, knowing the Memphis Express would be by in minutes, there was no time to lose. In a calm but serious tone, he instructed his son to stay put. Then, leaping to his feet, he ran to the bridge, ran up the catwalk, scurried up the ladder, and entered the control house.

Once inside, he searched the river to make sure no ships were in sight. Then, as always, he looked down beneath the bridge to make sure nothing was below. It was all routine. That is, till then. But in that moment, in that instant, something caught his eye. Something so shocking and so horrific he gasped in disbelief.

Trying to follow Dad, the boy had fallen off the catwalk and into the gears. With his leg now wedged between the two main cogs, he can't get loose. Twisting and turning, squirming and thrashing, he can't get loose!

John frantically searches for an answer as the train's whistle gets louder and louder. With heart pounding and mind racing, he looks all around, searching in vain. Lowering the bridge would be fatal. It'll kill his son, unless he can think of something and think of something fast.

In his mind's eye, he sees himself grabbing a rope, climbing down the ladder, running down the catwalk, securing the rope, sliding down to his son and pulling him to safety just in time to thrust down the lever. But the plan is futile, and John knows it. With the voice of reason screaming in his head, he knows there isn't time.

It's either save his son or save the 400 people aboard the train. And so, closing his eyes and gritting his teeth, John plunges down the lever. As his boy cries, "*Daddy! Daddy! Daddy!*" he plunges down the lever. But the cries are quickly drowned out by the relentless sound of the bridge grinding into place. With only seconds to spare, the Memphis Express crosses as scheduled.

The unthinkable horror of what has just happened is more than John can bear. Shattered beyond belief, he sobs uncontrollably as the train clears the bridge.

It's one of the most tragic stories I've ever heard, and reminiscent of another father and another son. The heart of God was broken as Jesus hung on the cross. He could have saved His Son but didn't. Knowing it was either Him or us, the Father looked away. As Jesus cried, *"My God, my God, why hast thou forsaken me?!"* the Father looked away. Sparing not His own Son, He delivered Him up for us all.

Chapter Twenty-Seven

Presidential Pardon Refused

CHRIST DIED FOR EVERYONE. So doesn't that mean *everyone* goes to Heaven? Wish that was true, but it's not. And here's why: God created us as free moral agents, which means we're free to choose. Consider George Wilson . . . .

On May 27th, 1830, Mr. Wilson was sentenced to death for armed robbery. But, having influential friends, great pressure was brought to bear on President Andrew Jackson to grant this man a pardon. The pardon was granted and, upon hearing the news, Wilson shocked the world. Most people would have been ecstatic under such circumstances, but not George Wilson. For some reason, Wilson refused the pardon and wanted to die.

This was highly unusual, had never been done. No one had ever refused a presidential pardon. And so, much debate ensued. Finally, the matter was brought before the U.S. Supreme Court and, in 1833, Chief Justice John Marshall announced: "*A pardon is a piece of paper, the value of which depends upon its acceptance by the person implicated thereon. It is unimaginable that one under sentence of death would refuse such a pardon. But, if refused, it is no pardon. Therefore, George Wilson must die.*"

Today there's a full and unconditional pardon with your name on it, issued by the King of kings and Lord of lords. But, as wonderful as this is, it's virtually useless. It's useless unless you accept it. "*Believe on the Lord Jesus Christ and thou shalt be saved . . .*" (Acts 16:31).

We could argue theology all day, but there's no rebuttal for a changed life. In the following pages you'll read of five people who were radically transformed through a personal encounter with the living Savior.

CHAPTER TWENTY-EIGHT

Gang Leader Trades Gun for Bible

HAVING PARENTS STEEPED IN WITCHCRAFT, Nicky Cruz was raised in a terrible environment where physical abuse was the norm. The abuse went on for years and, at the age of 15, he had had enough. So, with suitcase in hand, this young Puerto Rican fled the island and went to New York.

Once there, he moved in with his older brother and enrolled in school. But Nic's schooldays were short-lived. After cracking someone's skull open with a chair, he was expelled. Not for a day, not for a week, and not for a year, but forever. Which didn't sit well with his brother.

Nicky's brother was big on education and gave Nic an ultimatum. "*Either go to school or get out.*" So Nic got out. With no food, no money, and no coat, he got out. Having been expelled and evicted all in one week, this wayward child roamed the streets, looking for a place to stay.

After spending one or two nights in the subway, and committing his first armed robbery, Nic found a place. A one-room apartment in the projects with a panoramic view of the slums. Within a few days, he had joined a street gang and, within six months, had risen through the ranks and become its leader. Which was an enormous task for a sixteen-year-old.

Life in the gang was all-consuming, demanding his time and attention. But being the leader had its perks. Almost one-third of the gang members were girls, 75 to be exact, and Nic had his pick. What's more, he had first take of all that was stolen, which was usually enough to buy his food and pay his rent. And there were also the parties, the nightly bash with sex, drugs, and rock-n-roll.

But, aside from the girls and the parties, there were also the borders. And perhaps the gang's biggest job was guarding 'em, which meant confrontation. Rival gangs were always encroaching on each other's turf, trying to expand their own. So confrontation was par for the course and quickly turned into all-out war. Hand-to-hand combat.

Some had guns. Most had knives. A few had baseball bats or homemade clubs with a nail sticking out one end. Others had bicycle chains which proved lethal when swung at a boy's head. No doubt the weapons were crude but, crude or not, they did the job.

As leader of the most feared gang in the city, Nic was infamous and enjoyed the notoriety. The gang's reputation kept police at bay, and Nic's macho image attracted the ladies. All was well in gangland, or so it seemed.

Fast forward three years. Nic is now 19 and we find him and his cohorts sitting on the steps when a group of kids come running by at full throttle. "*Hey, where's the fire? What's goin' on?!*" shouts Nic. "*There's a circus down at the school,*" they reply. So Nic and the others follow. They follow the kids down to the schoolyard where a crowd has gathered. Almost 100 kids stand blocking the street.

Pushing his way to the front, Nic expects to see a show. He expects to see a circus. But there is none. No clowns, no tigers, no acrobats, no nothing. Nothing but a trumpet player standing on a fireplug playing *"Onward Christian Soldiers."* And the man keeps playing it over and over until another man appears.

The second man is tall and skinny with a black book in one hand and a hanky in the other. Climbing atop a piano bench, he stands to address the crowd. But the crowd won't let him. The hoots and hollers get louder and louder, making it impossible to hear. But the man persists. Not giving up, he begins to pray. With head bowed and eyes closed, he prays in silence.

Finally, the noise subsides. As things get quiet, the man opens the black book and begins to read, *"For God so loved the world that he gave his only begotten Son, that whosoever believeth in him, shall not perish, but have everlasting life."* Then, expounding on the text, he says God loves everyone everywhere, and demonstrated His love by sending Jesus to die in our place.

At the close of his message, the man says he wants to talk with all the gang leaders. That's when alarms go off in Nicky's head. This man of the cloth is invading their world, and Nic doesn't like it.

The man continues, *"If you're so big and tough, you won't be afraid to come up here and shake hands with a skinny preacher."*

After a long pause, someone calls out from the rear, *"Hey, Buckboard, whatsamatter, you scared?"* Buckboard is the leader of another gang, a black gang from the hood. There's a stir in the crowd and, looking back over his shoulder, Nic sees Buckboard and three of his gang members moving toward the front. They're walking toward the preacher, who has stepped down off the bench and stands ready to meet them.

After shaking the preacher's hand, they go with him and the trumpet player over to the doorway of the school. And, though Nic can't hear what they're saying, he can see. He sees what's happening and is stunned when all six of 'em get down on their knees. Removing their hats, Buckboard and his boys bow in prayer.

As the crowd disperses, someone shouts *"Hey, Nicky, you gonna let those niggers show you up? You afraid to go up too?"* Nic has no desire to go up, but the taunts continue. Then one of his own members yells, *"Hey, look at our leader. He's afraid of the skinny preacher!"*

There's no way, no how Nic is afraid of anyone, and I guess he has to prove it. So, working his way to the schoolhouse, he comes to the preacher and stands there. With hands in pockets and a piercing glare, he stands there.

Sporting a great big smile, the flamboyant preacher extends his hand, saying, *"Hi, Nicky, my name is David Wilkerson. I'm a preacher from Pennsylvania."* But Nic recoils, taking one step back. Then, after a moment of silence, he blurts out, *"Go to hell!"*

"I know you don't like me, Nicky," says the preacher, *"but I feel different about you. I love you. And not only that, Jesus loves you."*

As the preacher remains there smiling, with hand extended, Nicky trembles. He trembles in fear. Fear and anger. He fears this man might take his friends away and is angry about the same. *"You come near me, Preacher, and I'll kill you,"* says Nic as he turns and walks away.

Returning to the gang's hideout, Nic turns on the music, cranking it up as loud as it'll go. He's trying to drown out the words that keep ringing in his ears . . . . *"Jesus loves you."* Don't know why this bothers him, but it does. It bothers him.

When the music fails its mission, he thinks a bottle of wine might do the trick. So Nic starts drinking. Drinking, drinking, and drinking. But before passing out, or seeing sugar-plum fairies dance through the room, there's a commotion at the door. Someone has just entered the hideout. Someone unannounced, uninvited, and undeterred. Someone with nerves of steel and a God-given mission. And you're right, it's the preacher.

Walking across the room like he owns the place, he comes up to Nic, sticks out his hand again, and says, "*Nicky, I just wanna . . . .*" But, before he can finish his sentence, Nic slaps him and slaps him hard. He slaps him and spits in his face.

After a moment of stunned silence, the preacher says, "*Nicky, they spat on Jesus too, and He prayed, 'Father, forgive them; for they know not what they do.'*"

Screaming and yelling at the top of his voice, Nicky shouts, "*Get the hell outa here!*" as he pushes him back toward the door.

"*Nicky, before I leave, let me tell you just one thing: Jesus loves you.*"

"*Get out, you crazy preacher. You don't know what you're saying. You got 24 hours to get off my turf before I kill you.*"

The preacher backs out the door, still smiling. "*Remember, Nicky, Jesus loves you.*"

With anger and frustration, Nic grabs an empty bottle, smashing it to the floor. Never in his life has he felt so alone. But loneliness isn't something the gang talks about. Personal feelings and heartfelt emotions are somewhat taboo. So Nic plays along. The tough-guy image may be a farce but, farce or not, he plays along. If the gang ever knew his true thoughts and feelings, he'd lose their respect.

That night, he goes to bed early but can't sleep. Tossing and turning till 5 a.m., the preacher's words keep echoing in his mind. *"Jesus loves you, Nicky, Jesus loves you."* No one has ever loved him, not even his mother. So believing this Jewish carpenter could possibly care is a stretch. How could anyone love him after all he's done?

Getting up, Nic gets dressed, goes downstairs and sits on the steps. With head in hands, he sits there brooding. Brooding and thinking. And, as he sits, a hand is suddenly placed on his shoulder. Looking up, he sees the preacher.

"Hi, Nicky. Do you remember what I told you last night? I just wanted to come by and tell you again. Jesus loves you, Nicky."

Jumping to his feet, Nic takes another swing at the man, but this time he misses. Wilkerson ducked. Then looking Nic straight in the eye, he says, "*You could kill me, Nicky. You could cut me up into a thousand pieces and lay 'em all out on the street. But every piece would cry out, 'Jesus loves you.' And you'll never be able to run from that.*"

"*I'm not scared of you, Nic. You talk tough but, deep inside, you're like everyone else. Lonely and afraid.*"

This gets Nic's attention. "*How'd this man know I was lonely?*" Nic asks himself. "*I'm surrounded by girls and gang members every day of the week, so how could I be lonely?*" Bolstered with pride, he denies the obvious.

"*You think you're gonna change me just like that?!*" snapping his fingers in the preacher's face. "*You think you're gonna make me one of your converts?!*" Of course, Nic isn't wanting an answer, but hopes the sarcasm will drive him away.

The preacher continues, "*Nicky, you didn't sleep much last night, did you?*" Again, Nic is amazed. How'd this man know he hadn't slept? "*I didn't sleep much either,*" says the preacher, "*but stayed awake praying for you. Nicky, I've come to tell you that somebody cares. Jesus cares. He loves you. And one day soon, God's Spirit is gonna deal with you, and you're gonna stop running.*"

Without saying another word, Nic turns and leaves. He saw God's love in the preacher's eyes and didn't know *what* to say. Had the man attacked him with a gun or knife, he could have handled it. But how do ya deal with love?

In the coming days, Nic does his best to avoid the preacher, but the others won't shut up. Like fingernails on a chalkboard, the gang keeps talking about God. Finally, in a fit of rage, Nic shouts, "*Damn it! If you guys don't shut up about this God stuff, I'm gonna kill you!*" But they can't. They can't and they won't. They won't shut up.

It's the second week of July when one of 'em tells Nic about the preacher's big meeting down at the St. Nicholas Arena. The entire gang has been invited and, to ensure their attendance, the preacher has chartered a bus for the group.

Nic feigns indifference, saying he wants nothing to do with it, but succumbs to pressure when one of 'em asks if he's chicken. *"I ain't afraid of no one!!"* says Nic. *"Not you, not the preacher, not even God!! Just tell me when and where that bus will be picking us up and I'll be there!!"*

Wanting to prove his gargantuan courage, he's determined to show. But, determined or not, he dreads it. Remembering what happened to Buckboard and the others, he fears the same might happen to him.

When the day arrives, more than 50 gang members board the bus and, en route to the arena, they're shouting obscenities, smoking cigarettes, and drinking wine. Upon arrival, most of 'em exit through the emergency door and some climb out the windows.

Leading the pack, Nic takes his group to the main entrance but is quickly accosted. Thinking the service is much too refined for the likes of these hoodlums, an usher tries stopping them at the door. But the usher's blockade is no match for the gang, and the man stands helpless as they push their way through.

Finding their seats, Nic scans the crowd and, seeing other gangs there, he knows things could get ugly. The players are all present and the night could easily end with a full-scale riot.

But frivolity is in the air and everyone's much too busy mocking the meeting to mess with a riot. The place is a free-for-all, and Nic's gang joins in the whistling and shouting.

Sitting at the organ, a girl begins to play. That's when a kid in the crowd stands to his feet and, clutching his chest, shouts, *"Oh Jeeesus! Save my big black ass!!"* Then collapses in his seat amid the howls and the laughter.

Another girl takes the stage and, standing behind a microphone, begins to sing. But the noise is deafening and the poor girl can't be heard. *"Hey, babe, shake it a little!"* someone shouts. *"Hey, hun, how 'bout a date?"*

The girl is mortified but continues to sing. At least for a while. Trying her best, she starts singing louder. But the incessant catcalls and lewd remarks are taking their toll. As her voice begins to crack, she breaks down in tears and runs from the stage. That's when the preacher appears and, as he steps to the mic, a hush sweeps over the crowd.

The preacher begins to preach and, as he preaches, Nic remembers. He remembers his childhood and all the hate he's had for his parents. He remembers hitting that boy with the chair. He remembers getting expelled and joining the gang. He remembers the drugs, the girls, the fights, the parties. He remembers it all and knows that none of it has satisfied. None of it has filled the void.

"Christ died for our sins," says the preacher. *"He died for our sins and rose again. All the hell that you and I deserve, Jesus suffered on the cross. He suffered so that we won't have to. No matter who you are or what you've done, God loves you and wants to forgive."*

At the close of his message, the preacher gives an altar call, inviting those wanting to receive Christ to come forward. And, before he knows it, Nic finds himself at the front. He's at the front kneeling and crying, and isn't alone. Several of the others have also come forward and are kneeling there beside him. As he cries, Nic suddenly feels the preacher's hand on his back. *"Go ahead, Nicky, let it out. Pour it out to God. Call on Him."*

With eyes shut tight and tears streaming down his face, Nicky prays, *"O God, if you love me, come into my life. Come into my life and change me. Please change me. I'm tired of running."* And, as he prays, the burden is lifted. The burden of guilt.

When they all finish praying, the preacher shares 2nd Corinthians 5:17. *"If any man be in Christ, he is a new creation; old things have passed away and, behold, all things have become new."*

In his illustrious career as a gang member, Nic stabbed 16 people and was arrested 21 times. But that was the old Nic, and the old Nic is now dead and gone. The new Nic has just been born again.

Giving Bibles to everyone, the preacher shares words of encouragement. Each is assured their sins are forgiven, and all are encouraged to join a local church. The next day, they turn their weapons over to police and, in the days that follow, they begin reading their Bibles, attending church, and finding jobs.

It isn't long before Nicky feels called to the ministry. So, moving to California, he enrolls in Bible school where he meets his future bride. Bells ring, sparks fly, and Cupid glistens. It's a whirlwind romance, complete with goose bumps and all the feelings. But that, my friend, is another story.

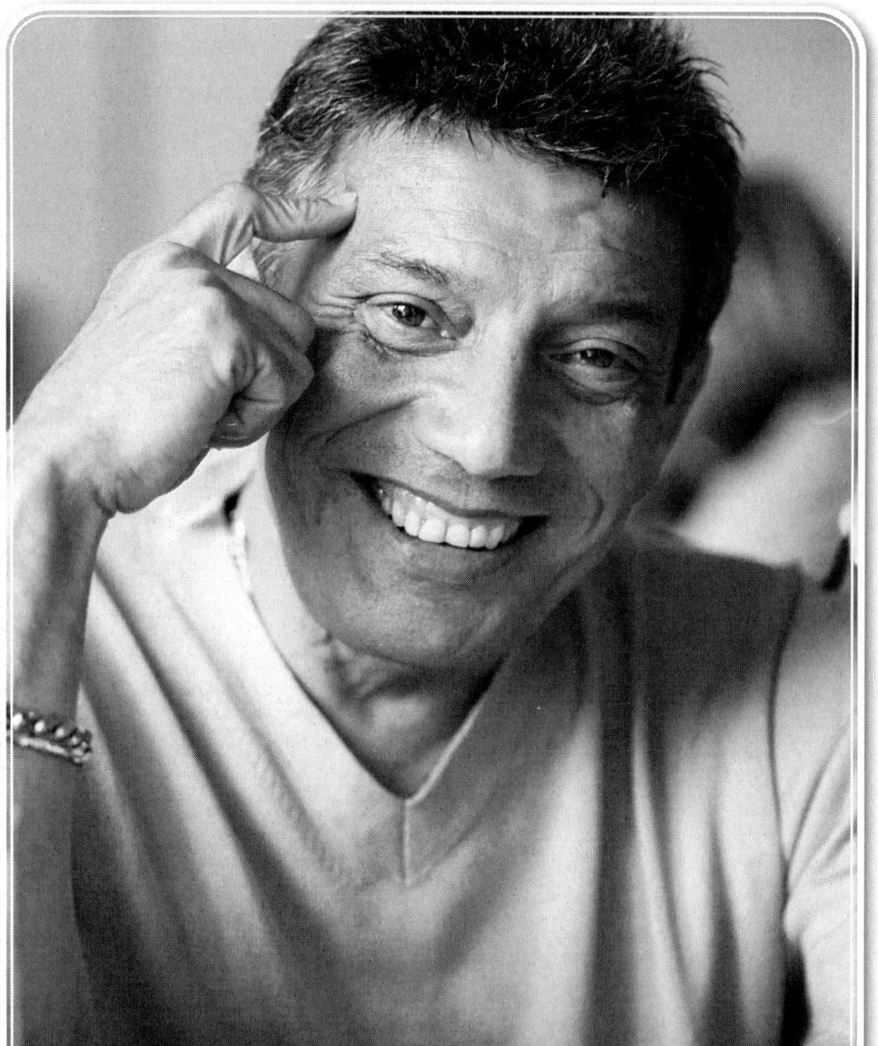

Nicky Cruz

CHAPTER TWENTY-NINE

Mafia Boss Quits Mob and Lives

IT HAS LONG BEEN SAID that the only way out of the Mob is in a pine box. So why is Michael Franzese still breathing? No, he's not the only one to quit, but he's the only one who quit and lived to tell about it. All the others are either dead or hiding out in the Witness Protection Program. But not Franzese. He's alive and well, living with his wife and kids in California.

So why is Franzese still living? Why hasn't he been whacked?? There are two reasons:

> #1 He's not a snitch. When arrested by the Feds, Franzese readily confessed to his own crimes but refused to turn state's evidence. Though doing so would have reduced his sentence, he wouldn't snitch.

#2 The Mob respects his faith. Franzese had become a born again Christian and, call it a hunch, my guess is that grand larceny and racketeering didn't mesh with his newfound faith. Thankfully, the Colombo family knew this was the case and let him walk.

However, Franzese didn't know it. He didn't know they'd let him walk. The day he turned his back on the Mob, he fully expected retribution. So yes, there was fear. But his faith in Christ was greater. Fear or no fear, he had to serve the Lord. Live or die, he had to serve the Lord.

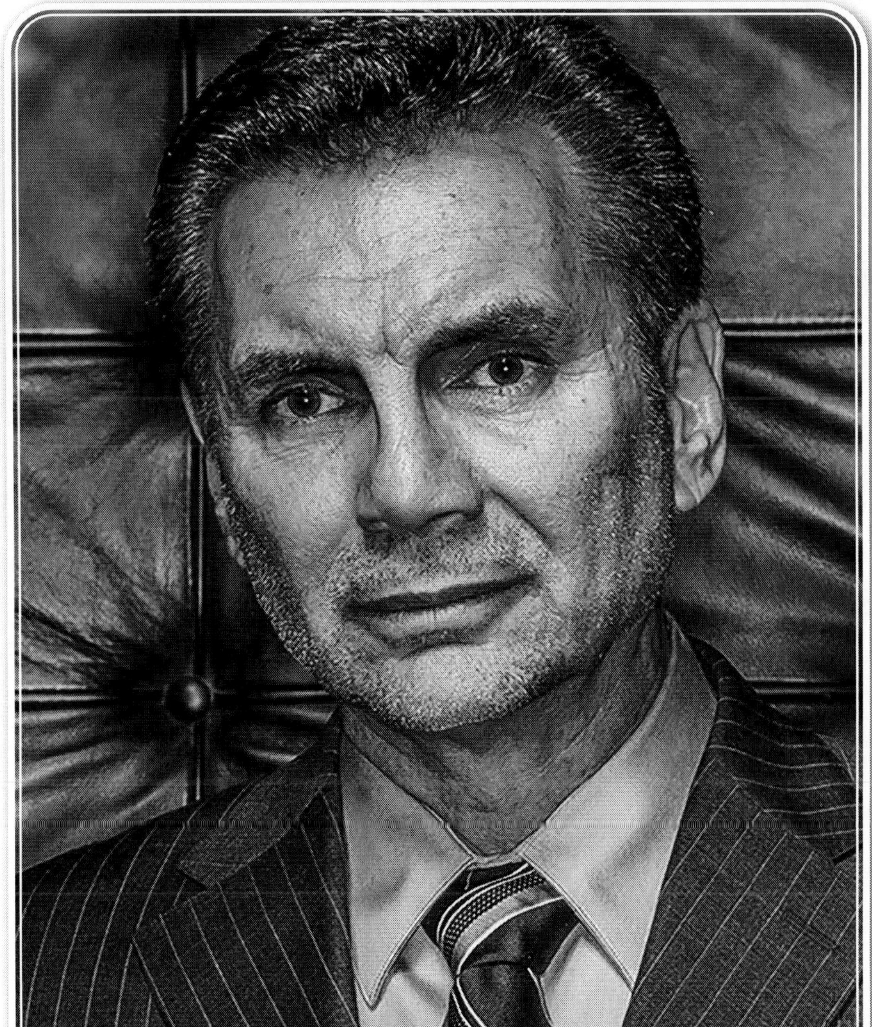

Michael Franzese

Chapter Thirty

Condemned Killer Forgiven

HAVING COMMITTED TWO MURDERS while high on drugs, Karla Faye Tucker was sentenced to die by lethal injection. And die she did. The execution was carried out on February 3rd, 1998. But the real story here is what happened in between. Between the events just mentioned.

It was during a weekend bash (a weekend of smoking cocaine, shooting heroin, and popping pills) that Karla and her live-in lover, Danny Garret, drove to Jerry Dean's apartment in hopes of stealing his motorcycle. They didn't expect Jerry to be home, but he was. And at 3:00 a.m., he and Deborah Thornton were asleep in the bedroom. That's when Karla and Danny entered the apartment.

The sleeping couple may have been awakened by the would-be robbers. But since that couple is now dead, and since Karla and Danny were high on drugs, no one knows.

I'll spare you the details, but knowing the media dubbed this as "*the pickax murders,*" well, you can imagine. With bloody fingerprints and footprints all around, the mystery was easily solved. Karla and Danny were soon arrested and brought to trial.

Testimony began on April 11th, 1984. But the Karla who testified in court that day was dramatically different from the woman who had committed this heinous crime. Though she had entered a not guilty plea during arraignment, she changed it to guilty and was willing to accept the outcome "*whatever it might be.*"

So what happened? What turned this cold-blooded killer into a repentant lady, a lady showing sincere remorse, a lady wanting to own up to her actions?

While awaiting trial, a prison ministry group had visited the jail. "*I just went to see what it was like,*" said Karla. "*They were putting on a puppet show. When I walked through the door, my mouth dropped open. I felt something that I had never felt before. I know now that it was the presence of God. I remember looking at the ministry team and knowing they had been where I was at. That they had been in jails and prisons. That they had been into prostitution, drugs, and violence. But still, they had this peace and joy. Something that was real. Something I had never seen before. I remember thinking, 'I want to feel what they're feeling.'*"

"*That night, when the service was over, I snuck a Bible. Didn't know they gave Bibles out freely to people in jail, so I thought I was stealing it. I took it with me to my cell and hid back in the corner. Then, opening the Bible, I started to read. Don't know how long it took, but I remember kneeling on the floor, crying, asking God to come into my heart and forgive me for what I had done.*"

"I don't know that I felt forgiven at that point, but I do know I felt loved. I knew that, no matter what I had done, I was loved. Just like that, just like I was. That's when the whole weight of what I had done fell on me. I realized for the first time that I had brutally murdered two people and there were people out there hurting because of me. Yet God was saying, 'I love you.' It was supernatural. I don't really know how to explain it. At that moment, He reached down inside of me, ripped out all the violence, and poured Himself in."

"I knew then that I had to tell the truth. Before I knew the Lord . . . I didn't want to tell what had happened for fear of consequences. But when the Lord came into my life and changed me . . . I had to tell the truth about everything."

Because of Karla's open confession, her conviction was swift, though the appeals process lingered on for 14 years. For 14 years, motions were filed and hearings were held. For 14 years, they tried getting her death sentence commuted to life in prison. The endless wrangling and contentious arguments went on and on but, in the midst of it all, Karla's attitude was always the same. *"If the Lord wants me to stay, I'll stay,"* said Karla, *"and if He wants me to go, I'll go. To die is gain."*

Death for the Christian is always a promotion, a promotion from this life to the next. And on February 3rd, 1998, Karla Faye Tucker was promoted. Escaping the bonds of the Huntsville prison, she stepped into Heaven and into the arms of Jesus.

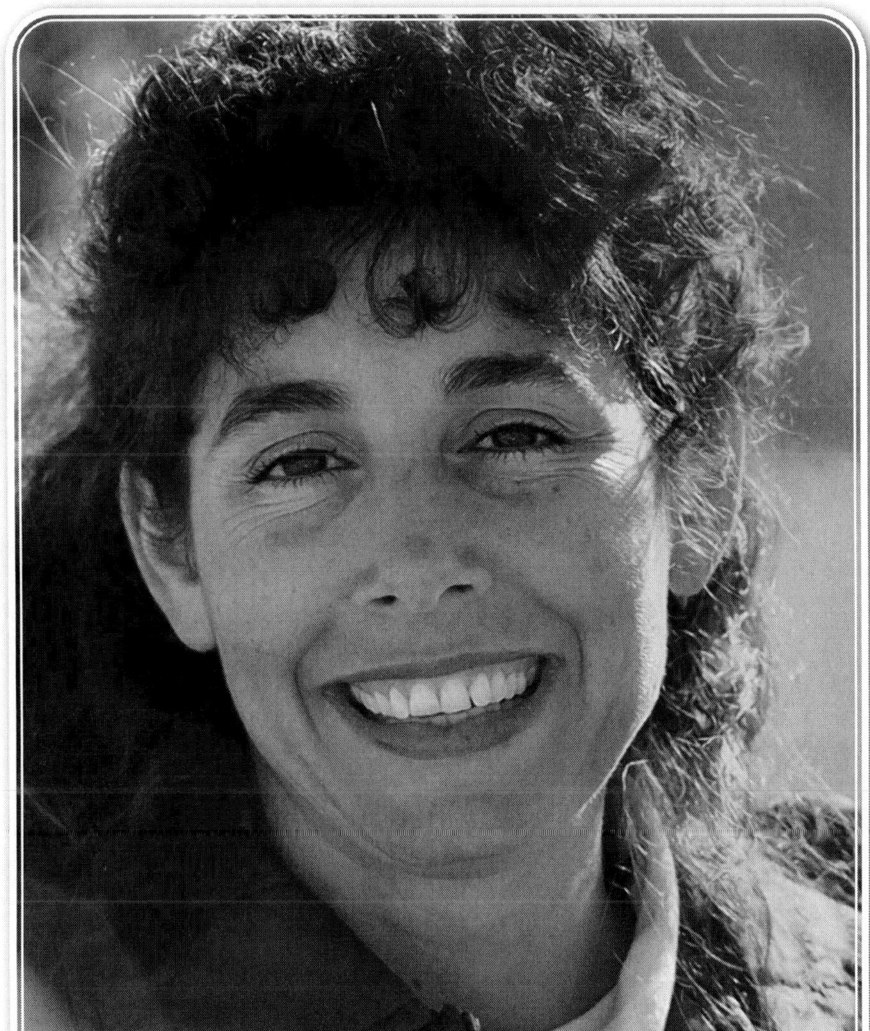

Karla Faye Tucker

Chapter Thirty-One

The King of Cool

THE WORLD KNEW STEVE McQUEEN AS AN ACTOR, but few knew of his personal struggles or the enormous void inside. A void that neither alcohol nor drugs could fill.

Having starred in films like *The Great Escape, Sand Pebbles,* and *The Reivers,* McQueen was well established as a cinematic icon and, by 1974, had become the world's highest-paid actor. But, despite the movies, money, and accolades, the void remained.

Like a runaway train, his fame kept growing, the scripts kept coming, and the crowds kept going. It was a box-office boom and the studios knew it. Everyone knew it. But the boom went bust when McQueen up and quit.

Turning his back on Tinseltown, McQueen walked away. At the height of his career, he walked away. Leaving the business to travel the country in search of answers, he knew there was more. There had to be more, more to life than making movies and signing autographs.

McQueen's departure was a major jolt to Hollywood insiders and was grieved by agents and fans alike. So you can imagine the elation when he returned five years later. He returned to acting but the search continued. The void remained and the search continued.

Little did he know that his relentless quest was coming to an end. The void would be filled, the questions answered, and all he'd been looking for would soon be found. Found at the Ventura Missionary Church in Ventura, California. That's where he received Christ as Savior and that's where his life was turned around.

Contrary to critics, Steve McQueen didn't *"get religion"* because of some doctor's report or grim prognosis. He had known the Lord for a full six months before the cancer came along. So no, it wasn't the cancer that brought him to Christ but intercessory prayer, a series of events orchestrated by God, and a clear presentation of the Gospel.

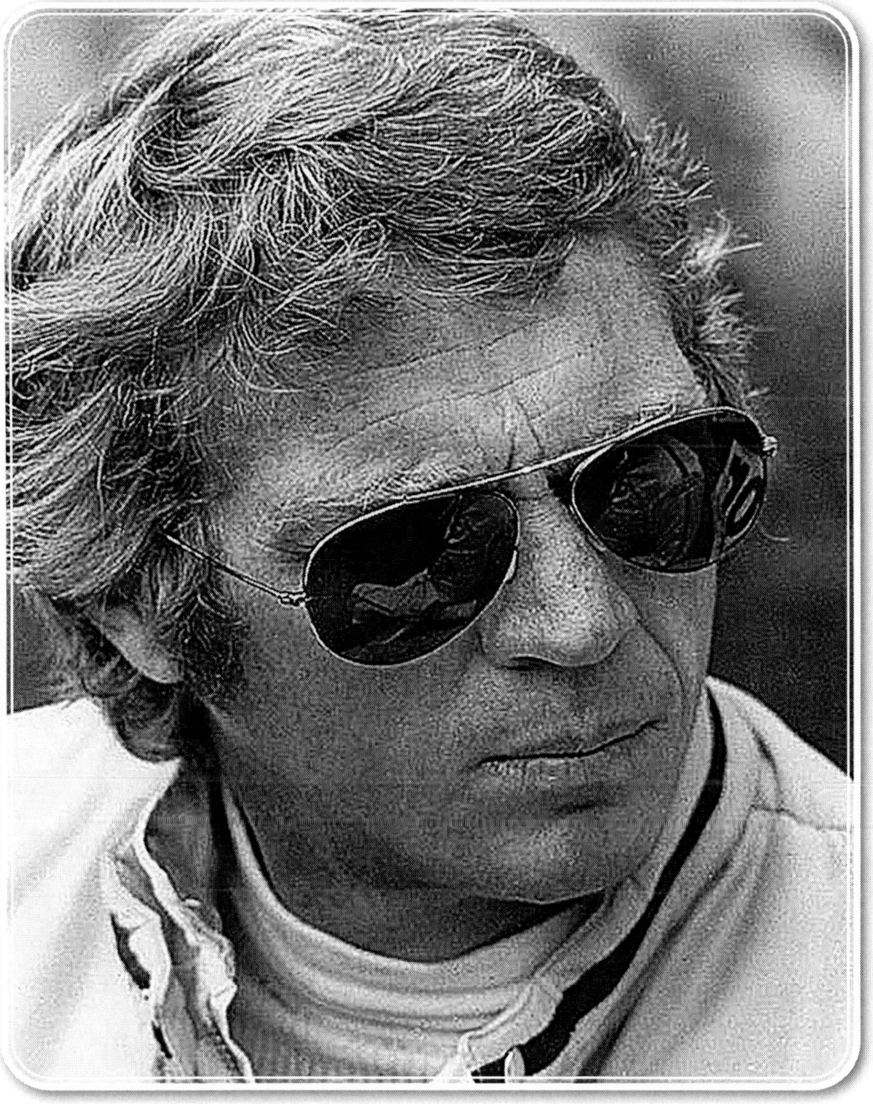

Steve McQueen

Chapter Thirty-Two

Surviving the Holocaust

AS A VIBRANT YOUNG JEWISH GIRL, Rose Price was full of joy and ready to take on the world. But the world wouldn't cooperate. Having been born in a time and place where Jews were despised, her hopes would fade and her freedom lost.

Coming from a close-knit family, Rose lived with her parents and sisters in Poland where the weekly Sabbath was a major event. "*Mother instilled in us that Judaism was life . . . and Shabbat* (Sabbath) *was celebrated as a holiday.*"

Every Wednesday, her mother and grandmother would start getting ready for the Sabbath, baking bread. Then, on Friday, they'd prepare the chicken, make the noodles, and take a cholent (a one-pot dish with meat, vegetables, and potatoes) to the baker to cook.

Meal time was family time, and fish was the dish on Fridays. *"When Father came home, he'd recite the blessing over the wine and the challa; then he'd bless the children."*

As dutiful Jews, they'd be at the synagogue each and every Saturday. After the service, they'd stop by the bakery, bring home the cholent, then sit around Grandmother's table and enjoy the meal.

The Nazi Horror

Change came quickly when Hitler took power. The Germans invaded in September 1939. Then, shortly thereafter, all the Jewish students were called up to the front of the classroom and, with guards standing by, they were told not to come back to school anymore. Rose was ten-years-old at the time, and was devastated.

The next item on Hitler's agenda was to evict the Jews from their homes and force them to live in the ghettos. The entire Jewish population of this small Polish town was corralled like cattle and forced to live on one street.

Then one day, as Rose and her sister were on their way to visit their grandmother, they were abducted. Suddenly and without warning, they were grabbed by Hitler's henchmen and forced to work in the ammunition factory, a dark damp environment where the hours were long, the beatings were constant, and conditions were freezing.

For a while they were allowed to return to their parents in the evenings, but this privilege was short-lived. Rose soon found herself confined to a prison camp 24/7. Both her and her sister. And, knowing they would never see their parents again, Rose cried. She cried and cried and cried. She cried till there were no tears left to cry.

At first she still prayed. Each morning she'd say the Modeh Ani, and during the day she'd say the Shema and just pray to God. One day she prayed that God would send her mother. "*I was hungry and homesick, and needed a mother's hug instead of the beatings. I prayed, but nothing happened. And when my prayers were not answered, I concluded there was no God.*"

What the Nazis did to these girls was unthinkable. Each morning, while still dark, they were drug from bed, pushed out the door, and forced to line up in the freezing cold. No matter how deep the snow, they'd stand in line for hours, half naked and without shoes.

One day, the Nazis had them line up completely undressed to see how long it would take for their blood to freeze. The only reason Rose survived this was because several of the others had passed out, falling on top of her, which kept her from freezing. Their body heat kept her from freezing.

Rose and her sister were transferred from one concentration camp to another until they arrived at Dachau, where the torture continued. Their daily rations consisted of a quarter-inch thick piece of bread, most of which was sawdust, and a cup of coffee. Hardly enough to exist on, let alone sustain someone working in extreme cold.

Being put in a field and forced to dig sugar beets out of an almost frozen ground with bare hands, their knuckles were busted and bleeding.

One day, determining that her belly was not going to hurt that night, Rose stole a sugar beet to eat. But was caught, and got such a beating that, even today, *"I can still feel the cat-o'-nine-tails on my back, on my face, and around my body. And I can still feel the pain from hanging by my hands."*

Twice, Rose was selected to be shot, but ran away when the guards unlocked her chains. The second time she ran into a guard, bouncing right off of him. And, believe it or not, the guard didn't notice. Had he noticed, had he seen her, he would have shot her himself. But, thankfully, the guard was oblivious. Oblivious to the bounce, oblivious to the cold, and oblivious to this girl as she fled for her life.

End of War

When they were finally liberated in May 1945, Rose was full of bitterness toward the Germans for all they had done and all she had been through. She hated them with a passion, and the hatred literally poisoned her body resulting in 27 operations.

She wanted someone to drop a bomb on Germany and Poland. Her sister and one aunt was all the family that remained. The krauts had killed all the others – nearly 100 relatives.

After being released, she moved to America, got married, and had children. And, though angry at God, she became active in the synagogue. "*My children needed to learn about Judaism, and I couldn't teach them because I was dead inside. Socially, I was the best Jew, helping to build the Hebrew school, and working my way up to become president of the sisterhood.*" But if someone had asked, "*Do you believe in God?*" she would have said, "*No.*"

Daughters Convert

One day when her teenage daughter announced that she had received Jesus Christ as her promised Messiah, Rose nearly had a heart attack and panicked. Telling her daughter all that Christ had done to her and her family, and why she didn't have many aunts and uncles, she tried her best to dissuade her. Over and over, the Nazis had told Rose that, because she killed Christ, He hated her and had put her into the camps to kill her.

She also recalled an incident from her childhood when, at the age of seven, a Catholic priest hit her in the head with a crucifix for the "crime" of walking on the sidewalk in front of his church.

So, for Rose, the mention of Jesus Christ, or any mention of the church, was unpleasant at best and the flashbacks were constant reminders. Which explains why her daughter's conversion to Christianity was deemed as the ultimate betrayal, and why her daughter was evicted from the home.

When Rose's husband went to check on their daughter at the house where she was staying, he too became a Believer. Had he known that house was being used as an evangelistic outreach, he may have avoided it altogether. But he didn't. He didn't know. He had no idea and, as an unsuspecting target, he entered the trap, emerging as a born again Christian. At least, that's how Rose would later describe it.

Though still attending a private Hebrew school, their youngest daughter also received Christ, and Rose beat her for it. Then, when her husband revealed that he had accepted the Lord, she disowned him.

She had lost her first family to the Nazis and now, it seemed, she was losing her second family to this Jesus. Knowing that both daughters had trusted in Christ was disturbing enough, but her husband's conversion sent her over the edge.

Rose was ready to leave the family. And, had it not been for the warning, she would have. Having been told that leaving the children could land her in jail, she decided to stay. Child abandonment is punishable by fine and imprisonment here in the U.S.

Since her husband had become a Believer, he insisted that their eldest daughter come back home, and she did. Their daughter came home, and she and her dad began witnessing to Rose. Time and again, Rose would find her Jewish Bible opened to certain passages, passages about Yeshua HaMashiach.

Counter Attack

Running to the rabbi, she asked for Jewish Scripture verses to counteract the verses her family was sharing with her. But, for every verse she countered with, they would give her five more.

At the urging of her daughters, Rose asked the rabbi about Isaiah 53, and the rabbi said, "*No Jew reads that passage, especially a Jewish woman.*" So she couldn't read it. And the same was true with Psalm 22. There are 328 prophecies concerning the coming Messiah and His sufferings, and Rose asked the rabbi about all of 'em, or almost all.

Finally, in violation of the rabbi's instruction, Rose read Isaiah 53, and was banned from the synagogue. In protest, Rose yelled at the rabbi saying, "*My family is dead because they believe in Jesus!! Help me!!!*" But the rabbi replied, "*No. I can't help you anymore.*" And so she returned home and began reading the New Testament. She'd sneak down to the basement, lock the door, and read the New Testament.

Starting with the book of Matthew, she learned that Jesus was a gentle man, and wasn't the killer of her people. He was very gentle.

The Millionaire

A short time later Rose went to a dinner at Arthur DeMoss' house. Mr. DeMoss was a wealthy Christian businessman who opened his home once a year as an outreach to Jewish people. While there, Rose was asked if she would mind him praying for her. She replied, "*You can stand on your head if you want, it's your house.*" But, instead of standing on his head, DeMoss led her in a simple prayer:

"God of Abraham, Isaac, and Jacob, if it's true, if Jesus is your Son, and if He's really the Messiah, please show me."

This was the first she had prayed since 1942, and the first she had cried since the war. An enormous weight rolled off her back and she felt so clean. She knew Christ was real and received Him as her Messiah.

From that day forth, the road was fraught with trials and temptations, but perhaps the biggest test was when an ex-Nazi asked her to forgive him. Her body shriveled up in pain as he knelt down before her, pleading for forgiveness. Then, suddenly, she realized this man had been a guard at Dachau, and you can't imagine the hell she suffered at Dachau. Part of her wanted to turn and run, but she didn't. She didn't run. Instead, she stood there and forgave him. Much to her own surprise, she forgave him.

CHAPTER THIRTY-THREE

Astronomical Odds

THERE ARE OVER 300 OLD TESTAMENT PROPHECIES concerning the first coming of Christ, all of which were fulfilled to the letter. But certain skeptics say this was nothing more than chance or coincidence. A mindless argument that was addressed by Professor Peter Stoner, Chairman of the Mathematics Department at Pasadena City College.

Citing the time of Christ's birth (Daniel 8 and 9), the place of His birth (Micah 5:2), the manner in which He was to be born (Isaiah 7:14), the fact that He'd be betrayed for 30 pieces of silver (Zechariah 11:12), that He'd be mocked, pierced, and crucified (Psalm 22), and that He would die among the wicked (Isaiah 53:9), Professor Stoner said, "*The odds of just eight such prophecies being fulfilled by chance are 1 in* 10^{17} *or 1 in 100,000,000,000,000,000.*" That's one in one hundred QUADRILLION!

This would be the equivalent of covering the whole state of Texas with silver dollars two feet deep, marking just one of those coins with a pocket knife, then mixing 'em all together with a thousand bulldozers and expecting a blind man to bend down and, on the very first try, find the ONE COIN that had been marked.

Take another eight prophecies from the 300 plus, add those to the list, and the odds are unfathomable, i.e., 1 in 10^{45} (1,000,000,000,000,000,000, 000,000,000,000,000,000,000,000,000). Seriously, it's easier to believe in Santa Claus and the Easter Bunny than to think these things just happened by chance.

Chapter Thirty-Four

Pinpoint Accuracy

IT'S AMAZING ENOUGH that God fulfills prophcy, but did you know there are at least two prophecies that not only predict future events but the exact day those events are going to happen? And, in fact, they already have. The events in question are now in the past and recorded in the chronicles of history.

Though he lived over 500 years before Christ, Daniel predicted the exact day Christ would make His triumphant entry into Jerusalem, and that day was April 6th, 32 A.D. And Haggai, living in that same time period (500 plus years before Christ), predicted the exact day British troops would enter Jerusalem, and it happened just as he said. The day was December 9th, 1917. That was the day General Allenby and his men defeated the Turks, conquering Jerusalem without firing a shot.

Neither Daniel nor Haggai had a crystal ball, but what they did have was divine revelation! If you know anyone who questions the veracity of these claims, have them study Daniel 9:24-27 and Haggai 2:15-18. They should read the text, review the commentaries, and search the net. And, as they do, they'll begin to realize that God knows exactly what's going to happen before it happens. He knows the end from the beginning and is never taken by surprise.

There's another day predicted in Scripture. The exact day of an event that has yet to happen. More on this later.

Chapter Thirty-Five

Left Behind?

SOME SPOUT VERSES like Revelation 21:7, saying that only the overcomer goes up at the rapture. Which is true. But, in all their spouting, there's a subtle implication. They imply that "overcomers" are some type of super saints, an ecclesiastical elite that excludes you and me. However, according to 1st John 5:4, every born again Christian is an overcomer. This means EVERY Christian goes up at the rapture.

Lest you think the backslidden Christian is left behind, remember Paul's words: "*. . . we shall ALL be changed, in a moment, in the twinkling of an eye . . .*" Keep in mind that, when Paul said these words, he wasn't talking to the Galatians or Ephesians, but to the Corinthians, the most carnal church in all the New Testament. So you can rest assured that, if the carnal Corinthians go up at the rapture, you will too. That is, if you're a Christian.

Many professing Christians won't be raptured because they've never been saved or born again. But all true Christians, those who have trusted in Christ as Savior, will exit this Earth, will soar through the air, and will meet the Lord in the clouds on that glorious day.

Chapter Thirty-Six

Armageddon

". . . the Lord gathered the kings of the Earth together into a place called in the Hebrew tongue Armageddon (Revelation 16:16)*."*

"And the seventh angel poured out his vial into the air; and there came a great voice out of the temple of Heaven, from the throne, saying, It is done. And there were voices, and thunder, and lightning; and there was a great earthquake, such as was not since men were upon the Earth, so mighty an earthquake, and so great. And the great city was divided into three parts, and the cities of the nations fell: and great Babylon came in remembrance before God, to give unto her the fierceness of His wrath. And every island fled away, and the mountains were not found. And there fell upon men a great hail out of Heaven, every stone about the weight of a talent: and men blasphemed God because of the plague of hail; for the plague thereof was exceedingly great (Revelation 16:17-21)*."*

"And I saw an angel standing in the sun, and he cried with a loud voice, saying to all the fowls that fly in the midst of Heaven, Come and gather yourselves together unto the supper of the great God; That ye may eat the flesh of kings, and the flesh of captains, and the flesh of mighty men, and the flesh of horses, and of them that sit on them, and the flesh of all men, both free and bond, both small and great (Revelation 19:17-18)*."*

"And I saw the beast and the kings of the Earth, and their armies, gathered together to make war against Him, that sat on the horse, and against His army. And the beast was taken and with him the false prophet that wrought miracles before him, with which he deceived them that had received the mark of the beast, and them that worshipped his image. These both were cast alive into a lake of fire burning with brimstone. And the remnant were slain with the sword of Him that sat upon the horse, which sword proceeded out of His mouth: and all the fowls were filled with their flesh (Revelation 19:19-21)*."*

"And I saw an angel come down from Heaven, having the key of the bottomless pit and a great chain in his hand. And he laid hold on the dragon, that old serpent, which is the Devil, and Satan, and bound him a thousand years, and cast him into the bottomless pit, and shut him up, and set a seal upon him, that he should deceive the nations no more, till the thousand years should be fulfilled: and after that he must be loosed a little season (Revelation 20:1-3).*"*

When a first grade teacher took her class on a field trip, visiting the local post office, the Postmaster astounded the kids with the wanted posters. While explaining that the men and women on these posters were wanted by the law, a little boy raised his hand. Acknowledging the boy, the Postmaster stopped in midsentence and said, *"Yes, son, what is it?"*

The boy asked, *"Are these bad men and women?"* The Postmaster replied, *"Yes, they are. And the police are trying to catch them."* But this just made the boy more curious and, raising his hand again, he asked, *"Why didn't you just keep 'em when you took their picture?"*

It's a funny story. Funny but true. And it makes me wonder why God doesn't just keep him. Why doesn't God leave Satan in the pit? As you know, Satan will be cast into the bottomless pit for a thousand years. But why limit it to a thousand years? Why doesn't God just leave him there? If I was God, I'd leave him there. But I'm not God, and aren't you glad?!

So what happens when Satan is released? After a thousand years of writhing in pain and plotting revenge, he'll be out for blood and it won't be pretty. See Revelation 20:7-10.

Chapter Thirty-Seven

Exact Day

THOUGH NO ONE KNOWS when the rapture will occur, Scripture tells us the exact day of Christ's return to Earth. It's a little known verse found in the Old Testament. And you'll also find it here:

TheExactDay.com

Epilogue

There's no amount of good you can do that'll make God love you any more than He does already. And there's no amount of bad you can do that'll ever make Him love you less. God loves each and every one of us, and loves us with all His heart. Always has and always will.

Thus saith the Lord, *"I have loved thee with an everlasting love . . ."* (Jeremiah 31:3).

"For God so loved the world that He gave His only begotten Son . . ." (John 3:16).

"God demonstrated His love toward us in that, while we were yet sinners, Christ died for us" (Romans 5:8).

"Herein is love, not that we loved God, but that He loved us, and sent His Son to be the atoning sacrifice for our sins" (1st John 4:10).

If you have enjoyed this book, please post a review on Amazon. And no, it doesn't have to be long. Two or three sentences should suffice. Positive reviews help boost the book's ranking, which results in added sales. Of course, if you didn't like the book, your review won't help the ranking. But constructive criticism is always good, and we welcome your input.

How To Post Reviews:

1. Log in to your Amazon account.
2. Go to the specific product page for the book you want to review and then select the book format you used. If you don't have a direct link to the book page, you can use the search box at the top of the page to help you. Remember that some books have more than one edition, or are available in more than one format (such as Kindle, audiobook, paper-back, hardback, etc.), so be sure to navigate to the page for the edition you want to review and then select the appropriate format.

3. Scroll down to the Customer Reviews section and click on the "*Write a customer review*" button.

4. On the next screen you will see the title of the book you want to review and next to it, five light gray stars. Rate the book by clicking on the appropriate number of stars you want to give the book. Your selection will turn the stars blue. Here's a guide to the number of stars you should give:

   1 = I hate it.
   2 = I don't like it.
   3 = It's okay.
   4 = I like it.
   5 = I love it.

5. A text box will appear below the stars. Here you will write or paste in the text of your book review. Then you can also add a headline for your review, if you wish. When you're done, press the "*Submit*" button.

6. You will see the message "*Thanks for your review of* [the book you reviewed]. *We're currently processing your review and we will email you at* [your email address associated with your Amazon account] *as soon as this is complete.*"

7. Check your email for a message from Amazon containing your book review. It will also contain a link to "*See your full review.*"

About the Author

With mentors like Dr. Jimmy DeYoung, Grant Jeffrey, and Dr. David Jeremiah, Mike has gleaned the best from the best and has boiled it down into this easy-to-read synopsis. Having a firm grasp of end-time events, he explains the rapture, deals with the Antichrist, and covers the tribulation. Then, bringing readers to the edge of their seats, he tells of the ultimate duel. It's God vs Satan, the Creator of the universe vs the Prince of Darkness.

For interviews and speaking engagements, Mike can be reached at Admin@PilgrimsPress.com

Made in United States
North Haven, CT
04 November 2026

21771711R00088